D0276425

HEALTH AND EMPOWERMENT

6

03

HEALTH AND EMPOWERMENT
Research and Practice

Edited by

Sally Kendall

PhD, BSc (Hons), RGN, RHV
Professor of Primary Health Care Nursing,
Buckinghamshire Chilterns University College,
Chalfont St Giles, UK

A member of the Hodder Headline Group
LONDON • SYDNEY • AUCKLAND

First published in Great Britain in 1998 by
Arnold, a member of the Hodder Headline Group,
338 Euston Road, London NW1 3BH

http://www.arnoldpublishers.com

© 1998 Arnold

British Library Cataloguing in Publication Data
A catalogue record for this book is available from the British Library

ISBN 0 340 69256 1

1 2 3 4 5 6 7 8 9 10

Production Editor: Rada Radojicic
Production Controller: Helen Whitehorn
Cover Design: Mouse Mat Design

Composition in 10/12pt Palatino by Phoenix Photosetting, Chatham, Kent
Printed and bound in Great Britain by J.W. Arrowsmith Ltd, Bristol

Contents

List of contributors

Margaret Gordon, Community Nurse Manager, Whiteabbey Health Centre, Newtown Abbey, Northern Ireland

Felicity Hepper, SHO Psychiatry, St Mary's Rotational Training Scheme, St Charles' Hospital, London

Sally Kendall, Professor of Primary Health Care Nursing, Centre for Research in Primary Health Care, Buckinghamshire Chilterns University College, Chalfont St Giles, Buckinghamshire

Sue Latter, Senior Research Fellow, Centre for Research in Primary Health Care, Buckinghamshire Chilterns University College, Chalfont St Giles, Buckinghamshire

Andrée Le May, Senior Lecturer, Department of Health Studies, Brunel University, Uxbridge, Middlesex

Helen Roberts, Co-ordinator of R&D, Barnardo's, and Honorary Research Fellow, School of Public Policy, University College, London

Ian Robinson, Director, Centre for Research in Health and Illness, Department of Human Sciences, Brunel University, Uxbridge, Middlesex

Annette Scambler, Tutor, Open University, and Honorary Lecturer in Sociology, University College, London

Graham Scambler, Reader in Sociology and Director, Unit of Medical Sociology, University College, London

Jackie Sturt, Primary Care Project Worker, Buckinghamshire Health Authority, Aylesbury, Buckinghamshire

Keith Tones, Professor of Health Education (Emeritus), Leeds Metropolitan University, Leeds

Introduction

Sally Kendall

The notion of empowerment has pervaded the discourse on health for the past 20 years or so. Most authors would agree that the origins of the idea that empowerment was somehow intrinsically linked with health can be traced back to feminism, the self-help movement and collective consciousness – ideology born of 1970s thinking (e.g. Anderson, 1996). Whilst such ideology originated from radical socialist thought, e.g. from critical social theory (see, for example, Habermas, 1972) in more recent times it has become part of the accepted rhetoric of right-wing conservatism. A shift in the interpretation of empowerment from one of collective responsibility to individualist notions of self-care and self-responsibility has been evident in the health care literature emanating from the Department of Health (Department of Health, 1990, 1991, 1992, 1998). There appears to be no doubt in the literature that the concept is political as well as grounded in group and individual work. The health-related literature, particularly that concerning nursing and health promotion, is strewn with references to the concept of empowerment and its relationship to health, healthy living and the health care services. Much time is devoted to analysing empowerment itself (Gibson, 1991; Rissel, 1994; Rodwell, 1996; Jacob 1996), the counter-concept of power (Sines, 1993; Gilbert 1995) and the application of these to professional models of health care practice. Inherent in these arguments is the underlying assumption that empowerment is of itself a 'good thing', and that by acting in an empowering way, health professionals will become more effective and people will become healthier. There are very few analyses of the way in which the process of empowerment can be practised or the outcome of empowerment identified. This book sets out to challenge the assumptions on which current discourse is based and to provide a series of examples from research and practice that have been subject to a critical analysis of both the process and outcome of empowerment. This has been attempted in the context of health care reform, where the boundaries between those being cared for and the carer in provision of services are becoming less well delineated, and where the idea of the 'consumer' of health care is in the ascendant. The extent to which rhetoric (from any government) matches the reality of people's experiences is of interest here because, no matter how often we call patients clients or consumers, they will remain patients until there is a shift in power relationships in practice, research and policy terms towards recognition of the inherent expertise of people. However, this provokes further questions along the lines of whether this is what people want from their health care (i.e. to be empowered). To what extent have they been consulted? What are the most effective ways of involving people in health care? Some of these questions are tackled implicitly or explicitly in the chapters that follow but, largely due to the impression which one gains of the lack of integration between research and political rhetoric, there are objections which remain fraught and unanswered.

Definitions of empowerment

Many definitions of empowerment have been cited, and some authors have attempted to arrive at their own definition based on an analysis of preceding published thought. Very few definitions in the existing literature are based on inductive research, thus contributing to the paradox that, whilst it appears to be a 'good thing', empowerment in health, at least, has not been thus validated by those who would be empowered. Some authors take as their starting point the World Health Organization's definition of health promotion, namely 'the process of enabling people to increase control over and to improve their health' (World Health Organization, 1986).

As Rissel (1994) has suggested, this implies a *raison d'être* for empowerment. As other definitions of empowerment reveal, the WHO approach to health promotion potentially embodies both the political and the individual, psychological dimension of empowerment. Thus increasing control over health could be defined in politico-structural terms as being in support of changes to welfare benefits or increasing a person's self-efficacy towards a particular health behaviour. These two dimensions of empowerment, as Rissel (1994) points out, are quite diverse and can be utilized by health policy-makers in quite different ways. For example, in the first instance, empowerment could be utilized by policy-makers to ensure that different voices and agendas are heard in the policy-making process. In the latter instance, people can be made to feel as though they are being given more control by the use of powerful and persuasive literature (e.g. literature on patients' rights) which has no real legal sway. In the worst-case scenario of both instances, manipulation by propaganda is possible, which is arguably in direct opposition to empowerment.

Rappaport (1984) defines empowerment as a process: 'the mechanisms by which people, organisations and communities gain mastery over their lives'. This definition captures the idea that empowerment is something which occurs within the individual or community, and is not a simple transfer of power from one to another. Gibson also embodies this in her definition: 'empowerment is a social process of recognising, promoting and enhancing peoples' abilities to meet their own needs, solve their own problems and mobilise the necessary resources in order to feel in control of their own lives' (Gibson, 1991, p. 359).

However, Gibson's analysis is presented in the nursing context, and whilst the emphasis is on enabling and facilitating from within, one does not feel a strong sense of the nurses' role in the political and structural domain of empowerment from Gibson's work. This raises the question of the extent to which the practitioners of health care should be the political advocates of the people, or whether it is more appropriate to practise empoweringly at the individual level, with which nurses have more traditionally allied themselves.

Rodwell, in her concept analysis of empowerment, does not add a great deal to our understanding of the dimensions of empowerment: 'In a helping partnership it [empowerment] is a process of enabling people to choose to take control over and make decisions about their lives. It is also a process which values all those involved' (Rodwell, 1996, p. 309).

Again, writing from a nursing perspective, Rodwell is overall more supportive of an empowering approach where notions of helping partnerships and mutual decision-making are more prominent than critical consciousness-raising or radical action. Conversely Skelton, whilst declining to offer a definition of empowerment, does explicitly argue that the opposing domains of empowerment do present a challenge to nurses, which may result in a shift in focus for nurses:

> Such a shift in focus will involve the political decision to act as citizens and to claim the right to press for rights on behalf of other citizens. Actions of this kind will need to take account of the political realities of the time, including the current emphasis on 'consumers.'
>
> (Skelton, 1994, p. 422)

However, Skelton's paper provides little substantive evidence that nurses either wish to shift their focus or are themselves empowered enough to shift from patient-focused care to a citizenship model of practice. Moreover, as Skelton does acknowledge, we do not know whether patients want nurses to act on their behalf in this way.'

Empowerment – research and practice

The chapters which follow in this volume identify many of the above issues and scrutinize the value of empowerment through the process of research and the implications for practice. An important theme that emerges is the research method itself – to what extent is research an enabling experience for the participants? How are people involved in the development of the research? Can participants be true collaborators when faced with the powerful position of the academic? Indeed, should researchers even attempt to present research in such a way?

Sturt's chapter on action research with a primary health care team examines many of these issues. It can be seen as an example of action research where the stated aim was to work collaboratively with the team in order to empower them to approach their health promotion practice in a more enabling and effective way with the practice population. Sturt describes the difficulties that she encountered with this research approach, as well as the outcomes which indicate that a facilitated approach to changing practice can have a positive effect.

The issue of professionals themselves being empowered as a group is raised in Sturt's work and also in Latter's chapter, which explores the health promotion practice of hospital-based nurses. This work is significant because hospital nurses have traditionally been a marginalized group, despite their numbers, often described as being dominated by medical power and disregarded by the nursing management hierarchy (e.g. Chavasse, 1992). Latter's interviews and observations of nursing practice illustrate overwhelmingly the power struggle which nurses have to face in the field of health promotion. Whilst Latter has not engaged in an explicitly collaborative research design, the interviews could be described as empowering in themselves, since they enable the nursing voice to be heard in an environment which, from the nurses' own accounts, is not usually the case. The dilemma for the researcher is then to find a mechanism to allow the voice of nursing to be heard in a management and political arena.

Latter's argument, one which has been proposed by previous authors, is that nurses can only practise in an empowering way with their patients when they are themselves empowered. Gordon also elaborates on this argument in her chapter on breastfeeding. Gordon writes from her perspective as a practising health visitor and breastfeeding trainer, in the context of a social environment (Northern Ireland) where the prevalence of breastfeeding is below average, which is largely explained by the social culture. Empowerment for Gordon is therefore concerned with changing professional attitudes and extending the values learned through a specific training programme to parents in Northern Ireland. Ultimately, Gordon's aim is to empower parents to make the choice of infant feeding which is best for their child – in some cases this may not be breastfeeding, but the decision will be based on knowledge and insight, rather than on acceptance of the social norm. Whilst Gordon's contribution stops short of the notion of empowerment extending to political advocacy by health professionals and critical consciousness-raising, it clearly provides a platform for further research in this area. The indications from her interviews with fathers are that breastfeeding is a gender issue which extends right into the decision-making arena. Who decides, for example, whether to provide facilities in a public building for women to breastfeed their babies? What are the priorities when new public buildings are being planned (car parks, video games)? Who is listening to the voices of women and children?

Roberts takes up the issue of children's voices in her chapter on childhood accidents. This raises important ideas about the relevance of children in healthy public policy and also in the research approach. Listening to children through interviews about the ways in which they have taken risks and avoided accidents in the past provided rich data which could then be used to collaborate with town planners to reduce road traffic accidents among children. The methodological problems of researching children are implicit in this study, and are taken up again by Hepper, Kendall and Robinson in their discussion in Chapter 7 on conducting ethnography with children. The ethical and methodological complexities of observing and talking to children may be empowering in themselves or, as is more often argued, could lead to the accusation that the powerful researcher is making inappropriate interpretations of children's activities and life-views. The use of ethnography to explore the management of childhood asthma in a primary school provides the context for the argument that there are hidden opportunities to empower children which can be revealed through ethnographic approaches.

Other marginalized and potentially vulnerable groups are the subject of Le May's chapter, which explores communication with older people, and Scambler and Scambler's chapter, which takes a more sociological perspective on the health of women sex workers. Older people are becoming the subject of increasing attention in the health research literature since the introduction of the NHS and Community Care Act (Department of Health, 1990). When the Community Care part of the Act was introduced in 1993, the division between health and social care for older people in the community became an issue of concern for practitioners, health care managers and social workers, as well as for policy researchers. Criticisms were based on the fact that false and unfair decisions were being made on behalf of older people about what constituted health care and what was deemed to be social care. Bathing and dressing were examples of activities which could be classified as social care and had previously been carried out by community nursing staff. Under the Act, such activities were carried out by care assistants with no nursing experience. The significant factor in terms of empowerment is that little was done to take into account older people's views when these policy changes were implemented. Le May addresses the variety of ways in which communicating with and listening to the voices of older people, both at an individual level and on a community level, may enable their needs to be more appropriately analysed and understood. However, from the outset Le May also challenges the notion that older people need to be empowered, suggestive of the argument that to impose the rhetoric of empowerment on certain groups may in itself be undermining people's existing skills and attributes.

Similarly, the health needs of women sex workers are critically analysed by

Scambler and Scambler in the context of what in some ways may be described as a powerful group of women (prostitutes or sex workers) being marginalized with regard to their access to and the distribution of health services.

The extension of empowerment into public health policy is a significant theme if the ultimate and logical conclusion of the concept is to be operationalized. Tones, in Chapter 3, describes empowered communities as being made up of empowered individuals. This pervasive and persuading discussion provides much of the theoretical basis for empowerment within this volume. Tones' work on health promotion involves over 25 years of research and analysis of theories and concepts. It is therefore appropriate that a volume which aims both to contribute to the empowerment debate and to challenge some current thinking should draw on this considerable breadth and depth of experience. Some of the studies presented in this book draw significantly on the ideas of prevention, health promotion and radical action to enhance the possibility of empowering participants in their quest for health. The fundamental construct of self-efficacy as first described by Bandura (1977) is, for example, seen by Tones to be a prerequisite for empowering the individual units within an empowered community. Sturt has specifically analysed self-efficacy theory and its relevance to health promotion theory and practice. The outcome of this study is fascinating for those interested in either self-efficacy *per se* or its application . However, as Jacob (1996) has argued, there are objections to theories of empowerment which tend to advocate in terms of control and mastery. Feminist analyses may take a more interdependent approach. The more radical approach to community action has been considered by Roberts and also by Scambler and Scambler, and these studies provide real examples of a community approach, rather than the theorizing which it can so easily become.

With the publication of the consultation document *Our Healthier Nation* (Department of Health, 1998) at the time of this book being written, it is to be hoped that there will be new opportunities for community action. Certainly, the proposed Health Action Zones, in which it is expected that multi-agencies will work towards better health in defined localities, are a step away from political rhetoric towards restructuring the environment for health promotion. Throughout the document there is a much greater sense of 'involvement' for both consumers and professionals than has been the case in the past and client groups that were previously underrepresented (older people, children, for example) have greater prominence. All of the chapters which follow make a significant contribution to the way in which empowerment for health could lead to a healthier nation within current ideological thought, provided that the structural requirements meet with the reality of the changes which may yet be necessary to produce major shifts in health.

It is these integrating notions of empowerment which I have found persuasive in the final analysis of the debate surrounding empowerment.

Whilst political theory and rhetoric oscillate between individualism and collectivism, the real tenets of an empowering approach to health care appear to be grounded in the views and experiences of participants. However, each chapter exists in its own right and each author expresses his or her views, so ultimately it is left to the reader to decide whether empowerment is a valid and effective approach to practice.

References

Anderson, J.M. 1996: Empowering patients: issues and strategies. *Social Science and Medicine* **43**, 697–705.

Bandura, A. 1977: Self-efficacy: toward a unifying theory of behaviour change. *Psychological Review* **84**, 191–215.

Chavasse, J.M. 1992: New dimensions of empowerment in nursing and challenges (guest editorial). *Journal of Advanced Nursing* **17**, 1–2.

Department of Health 1990: *The NHS and Community Care Act*. London: HMSO.

Department of Health 1991: *The Patient's Charter*. London: HMSO.

Department of Health 1992: *The Health of the Nation – a strategy for health for England*. London: HMSO.

Department of Health 1998. *Our Healthier Nation*. London: The Stationery Office.

Gibson, C. 1991: A concept analysis of empowerment. *Journal of Advanced Nursing* **16**, 354–61.

Gilbert, T. 1995: Nursing: empowerment and the problem of power. *Journal of Advanced Nursing* **21**, 865–71.

Habermas, J. 1972: *Knowledge and Human Interest* (trans. J.J. Shapiro). London: Heinemann.

Jacob, F. 1996: Empowerment: a critique. *British Journal of Community Health Nursing* **1**, 449–53.

Rappaport, J. 1984: Studies in empowerment: introduction to the issue. *Prevention in Human Services* **3**, 1–7.

Rissel, C. 1994: Empowerment: the holy grail of health promotion? *Health Promotion International* **9**, 39–47.

Rodwell, C. 1996: An analysis of the concept of empowerment. *Journal of Advanced Nursing* **23**, 305–13.

Sines, D. 1993: Balance of power. *Nursing Times* **89**, 52–5.

Skelton, R. 199: Nursing and empowerment: concepts and strategies. *Journal of Advanced Nursing* **19**, 415–23.

World Health Organization 1986. *Ottawa Charter for Health Promotion: Conference on Health Promotion, 17–21 November 1986*. Copenhagen: WHO Regional Office for Europe.

PART I
Empowerment of professionals

1

Health promotion in the acute setting: the case for empowering nurses

Sue Latter

Introduction

In this chapter, findings from a recent research study are reviewed which suggest that an important relationship exists between nurses' ability to promote the health of patients/clients and the extent to which they themselves experience empowerment. It begins with an overview of recommendations regarding nurses' health promotion practice in acute settings, and reviews the calls made for empowering nurses. The author's own research, together with the work of others in this field, is then presented in order to illuminate the relationship between nurses' health promotion potential and nurse empowerment. Strategies which support the empowerment of nurses in the acute setting are presented and explored. The chapter concludes with a consideration of the challenges involved in achieving this goal.

In recent years, health and social trends have led to an increased emphasis on health education and health promotion. These include changes in patterns of morbidity and mortality, increased longevity, a political ideology emphasizing competitiveness within a market system, a rise in consumerism and calls for deprofessionalization. It has been suggested that nurses have a leading role to play in the health promotion movement (World Health Organization, 1989), and the importance of this role is reflected in nursing policy documents issued over the past decade (United Kingdom Central Council for Nurses, Midwives and Health Visitors, 1986; Department of Health 1989, 1993; Royal College of Nursing, 1989). Whereas traditionally health promotion was perceived as the territory of nurses working in primary health care settings, more recent recommendations focus on the need for all nurses, including those in acute sector hospital practice, to fulfil their health promotion potential. Nurses have the opportunity to develop relationships with patients/clients as a result of their intimate and continuous contact with them. Health and illness issues and experiences provide the focus for these contacts, and this may create particular opportunities – as well as particular constraints – for promoting health. Rodwell (1996), for example, highlights the potential contribution that nurses could make, suggesting that they are firmly placed in a position of close contact with health care consumers and could therefore make a significant impact on the lives and health of many individuals.

The concept of health promotion

Health promotion actions include establishing policy and legislation conducive to health, lobbying and advocacy, community development approaches, the provision of preventative services, and education for health at the level of the individual. As Macdonald and Bunton (1992) point out, there is now widespread agreement that health promotion combines the dual approaches of structural change on the one hand, and individual education for lifestyle change on the other. The form of activity chosen will depend, amongst other criteria, on situational factors, and it is intended that they are complementary. The nature of hospital-based nurses' practice indicates that their greatest (although not exclusive) contribution to health promotion may lie at the level of health education within the individual nurse–patient interaction.

There have been numerous attempts to describe approaches to, or models of, health education. For example, Rawson and Grigg (1988) identified at least 17 different taxonomies of health education models in an overview of the relevant literature. Despite this diversity, some common themes emerge from the literature which can serve as a quality framework for nurses' health education practice. A number of authors (e.g. Downie *et al.*, 1990; Tones and Tilford, 1994; Williams, 1995) highlight the need to move from a prescriptive, medical model, behaviour change approach, to one which aims to empower individuals with regard to health issues. Central principles include the need for two-way communication, partnership and collaboration, a requirement to clarify the patient's or client's beliefs, experience and values, and the importance of fostering self-esteem and self-efficacy.

Recently, Cribb and Dines (1993) have suggested that health promotion might also be defined according to whether an action is carried out in a health-promoting way. They argue that health-promoting actions are distinguished by the characteristics of holism, equity and collaboration. Macleod Clark (1993) has also developed the idea of defining an interaction as 'health nursing' by virtue of its process characteristics, as opposed to content or outcome measures. She outlines the need for interactions to be collaborative, individualized, negotiated, supportive and facilitative, as opposed to 'sick–nursing' interactions, which are nurse-dominated, generalized, prescriptive, reassuring and directive. Health–nursing interactions are more likely to be empowering for the patient or client, and are not necessarily confined to those with an obvious health education or lifestyle content, but can incorporate any interaction between a nurse and a patient or client.

In the light of the above, these concepts can be applied to hospital nurses' practice as follows:

- *health promotion*: an overarching term which refers to the whole range of activities possible, from nurses' engagement in both structural change activities, e.g. the creation of healthy hospital policies such as healthy menu choices and leisure areas, to health education interactions with patients/clients and also health-promoting nursing or health nursing, as outlined below;
- *health education*: refers to nurses' involvement in interactions with individual patients/clients which have an obvious health- and education-related content. Examples include education about medication, teaching self-care skills such as inhaler technique or urine testing, and giving preparatory information prior to a procedure. These interactions can be conducted according to either a traditional, prescriptive, behaviour change approach, or in line with an empowerment model of health education, characterized by such features as partnership, individualization and fostering the patient's/client's self-esteem and self-efficacy;
- *health-promoting nursing/health nursing*: refers to an approach to any interaction which is characterized by the features outlined by Cribb and Dines (1993) and Macleod Clark (1993). For example, these interactions are holistic, individualized and collaborative. The concept of health-promoting nursing/health nursing does not only apply to interactions with an obvious health- and education-related purpose, and may include, for example, interactions with the patient/client during a bedside handover, whilst updating care plans or preparing a patient for discharge.

The importance of nurse empowerment

Clearly, then, a fundamental aspect of nurses' health promotion role in acute settings is to engage in interactions with patients/clients in a manner which involves relinquishing power and control over them, and which instead facilitates their empowerment. Simultaneously, it has been suggested that facilitating empowerment in others requires the empowerer to have undergone a process of personal empowerment. This idea was proposed by Freire (1968), and has been applied in the nursing context by, for example,

Clay (1992), who suggests that it is necessary to empower nurses in order for them to empower the people who they serve. More recently, in her discussion of the transference of power involved in the process of empowerment, Rodwell (1996) also asserted that nurses cannot empower unless they themselves are empowered. Others (Lask, 1987; Watts, 1990; Clarke, 1991; Tones, 1993) have also argued that nurses need to be empowered in order to fulfil their health promotion potential. For example, Clarke (1991) states that with regard to the issue of nurses as healthy role models, individualistic victim-blaming is no more relevant to nurses than to others. She argues that just as important as observable good health behaviours in nurses is the development of strong self-image and confidence, and that the skills needed revolve around internal mechanisms and self-sentiment rather than external health behaviours. Tones (1993) proposes a similar argument, suggesting that any policy designed to achieve a health-promoting hospital should take account of the fact that a hospital consists of a community of both patients and staff. Consequently, he argues, its concern should be to empower not only patients but also staff, and in doing so nurses could effectively act as role models for empowerment. Other writers (Dalton, 1990; Weinstein, 1991; Carlson-Catalano, 1992) have extended this line of argument beyond the nurse's health promotion role, suggesting that empowerment is a necessary precursor to enable the development of professional practice by nurses.

Despite these recommendations, it has been suggested that nurses are not fulfilling their health promotion role, and that they do not experience empowerment, either individually, or as a group. For example, research by Johnston (1988) involved interviews with a randomly selected sample of 50 patients on surgical wards within one hospital. A singular lack of healthy lifestyle advice from nursing staff was reported by patients. However, the study concentrated on lifestyle advice only, and was exclusively concerned with patients' perceptions. Other studies by Macleod Clark *et al.* (1990) and Kendall (1991) have included observation of nurses' practice, and found that this is limited and lacking in a participatory approach. However, both studies focused on one particular aspect of the nurse's role in health promotion (smoking cessation advice and client participation in health visitor encounters, respectively), and the practice of hospital nurses specifically was not addressed. In addition, despite claims that nurses do not experience empowerment (e.g. Benson, 1991), there has been little research on this phenomenon in the practice setting, and its relationship to nurses' ability to promote health. The study described below set out to explore nurses' health promotion practice in acute care settings, and to identify the influences which impact upon this. One of the key findings to emerge was a relationship between nurses' own experience of empowerment and their ability to empower patients/clients as part of their health promotion role.

The study[1.1]

A qualitative approach was employed in order to generate in-depth data and meaningful insights into nurses' health promotion practice. More specifically, a case study design was selected, with individual wards selected as the unit of analysis. A multiple case design was used which enables constant comparison of settings, providing richness of data and important insights for theory development (Field and Morse, 1992). Three wards were selected as case studies of practice, from a sampling frame derived from a previous interview survey of ward sisters' views of health promotion practice on their respective wards (see Macleod Clark *et al.*, 1992).

A number of different methods of data collection were employed on each case study ward to enable a more complete picture of practice to emerge than would have been possible with the use of one method alone. This also enabled the 'between' method of triangulation to be employed which is where, according to Duffy (1987), data is collected by more than one method in order to determine whether there is convergence in the findings. The following methods were employed.

1. *Non-participant observation.* After gaining informed consent from relevant nurses and patients, a small group of four or five patients in close proximity to each other were selected for a 2-hour observation period together with the one or two nurses who had responsibility for their care at the time of observation. The method of recording the observations followed an essentially unstructured format, allowing an overall description of nurses' activities and interactions to emerge. Detailed verbatim description was devoted to any interaction that could be considered to constitute a health education-related interaction with a patient. Later, observation notes from each ward were analysed using a form of content analysis with a view to identifying the types of activities and interactions that nurses were engaged in, as well as the process or approach involved.
2. *Audio-recordings of interactions.* Various events and conversations on each ward were recorded using a hand-held tape-recorder. Given that the features believed to characterize an empowerment approach to health education and health nursing are rooted at the level of communication between individuals, it was essential to record conversational data in this way. Recordings included patient admissions, shift handovers and discharge advice, as well as planned conversations identified by the nurses as being of relevance to health education, e.g. educating a patient about medication or details of his or her diagnosis. Following transcription, notes were made about each interaction with a specific focus on the following: the types of health education activity involved (e.g. preparatory information-giving, advice on lifestyle); the approach taken (e.g. nurse-dominated, prescriptive or individualized and collaborative) and opportunities for health education that were taken or missed by the nurse.

Analysis of these notes provided an overview of recurrent themes pertinent to each ward.

3. *Post-observation interviews with nurses*. These required reflection on interactions characterized by principles of good practice (as described above) that had been observed. As examples of such practice were not found on two of the case study wards, only a small sample of nurses on one ward were interviewed in this way. Interviews were tape-recorded, transcribed and later analysed to illuminate perceived influences on practice from the nurses' perspective.

4. *Field notes*. These were made daily by the researcher, and involved the elaboration of key points jotted down as an *aide-mémoire* during the time spent on the ward. Field and Morse (1992) suggest that field notes represent both a data-gathering and an analytical tool to assist in understanding the phenomena under study and the setting or context in which those phenomena are occurring. In this study, field notes were used as a vehicle for gathering data about many informally observed events and conversations witnessed during the course of each day's data collection. In addition, they included an analytical element, allowing the researcher to record his or her thoughts about practice on each ward and the influences involved in this.

A detailed description of checks on reliability and validity is beyond the scope of this paper (see Latter, 1994). However, a variety of approaches were used, including sharing of data analysis with participants and expert nursing colleagues, in addition to utilizing the process of triangulation referred to above.

Data collection took approximately 4 weeks on each case study ward, and resulted in the following.

Ward 1: 7 periods of non-participant observation;
         7 recorded interactions.
Ward 2: 9 periods of non-participant observation;
         9 recorded interactions;
         6 post-observation interviews.
Ward 3: 8 periods of non-participant observation;
         11 recorded interactions.

Rather than imposing a fixed time for data collection or stipulating certain amounts of data, these were determined by the researcher's sense of the completeness of the picture of practice. That is, data collection ceased when no new data appeared to be emerging from each ward.

Findings

Nurses' health promotion practice

Analysis of the data sources revealed differences between the wards in the extent to which nurses' practice approximated the features of an empowerment model of health education or health–nursing interactions, characterized by the features described above.

On Ward 1, any form of health education was largely absent from the data collected and analysis indicated that nurses' interactions with patients did not accord with central health-promoting features. Comparison of the data from separate periods of data collection as well as between method triangulation repeatedly confirmed this finding. Both non-participant observation notes and recorded interaction data revealed that the only activity which could be considered to resemble health education was the practice of minimal information-giving to patients. However, even this appeared to be driven by the nurses' need to complete a task or activity with a patient. For example, nurses were observed to name a drug as they handed this to the patient during a drug round, whilst another nurse was observed informing a patient that she was now going to do his dressing. Nurse domination and a lack of collaboration and participation with patients emerged as a theme permeating both the recorded interaction data and the researcher's observations in the field notes. Patients' knowledge and expertise did not appear to be either sought or valued by nurses. This is exemplified by the following extract taken from a bedside handover:

Nurse 1 (1):	*I think we're just going on to test your urine. X explained about testing the urine, didn't she?*
Patient:	*I normally do that at home.*
Nurse 1 (1):	*You do that at home.*
Patient:	*Yes.*
Nurse 1 (1):	*Fine.*
Patient:	*I do that at home.*
Nurse 2 (1):	*Right, OK. So we'll be doing that twice a day now.*

In general, bedside handovers were characterized by a lack of collaboration with patients, and nurses spoke over patients in instances where there was no obvious reason why patients could not contribute. The following patient handover was typical of many:

Nurse 2 (1):	*Mr X has oedematous feet . . . it's still sore now and then. The majority of the time he's been sitting down here, while he was on the ward. He went off to get his barium enema today and hence the reason . . .*
Nurse 1 (1):	*He's not keen to keep them up at all.*
Nurse 3 (1):	*He finds it really difficult, don't you, keeping your legs up?*
Nurse 1 (1):	*I know, he's fed up with me . . . I'm sorry.*
Nurse 2 (1):	*He went off to get his barium enema today, and he's much better now. He's going to eat and drink. He didn't really have anything much today.*

All of the data sources revealed a lack of evidence of interactions that were potentially empowering for patients. Indeed, it is likely that interactions of the above variety were likely to be disempowering for patients.

On Ward 3, similar findings emerged from each of the various forms of data collection employed to allow some conclusions to be drawn about the characteristics of nurses' practice. The main health education activity on this ward took the form of preparatory information-giving to patients, and this was evident from observation notes, recorded interactions and field notes. This was usually associated with certain events, such as the admission procedure or sessions preparing a group of patients for discharge, as opposed to being responsive to individual patient need. In addition, tape-recorded data indicated that these interactions were not usually congruent with a health-promoting or empowering approach. Numerous examples revealed a nurse-dominated, standardized approach to giving information, rather than a stance which was individualized and collaborative. The following extract, taken from a recording of discharge advice being given to a group of patients, is illustrative:

Patient: *I'm just worried about my diabetes.*

Nurse 4 (3):   *Your diabetes, yeah. That's* (referring to an information sheet) *just a guideline really as to what are the best foods to eat really for a high fibre diet. You'll find your bowels will settle down in a few weeks and get back to normal again. Don't increase your fibre too much, otherwise you'll end up going to the other extreme and getting diarrhoea, but it is preferable to eat high-fibre foods really . . . to regulate your bowels. So if you just read that through and take it home. Can't think of anything else. If you do get any discomfort do take some paracetamol when you get home. You can have it four-hourly, but you're not to have more than eight in a day, because that's your safe dose in a day, only eight tablets a day, so try and space them out with your meals at breakfast, lunch, tea and supper, and it should be alright . . .*

The interaction continues in this manner for several more minutes. Whilst it may be difficult to cater for individual patients' needs in a group situation, this patient's concern about her diabetes is clearly not addressed by the nurse, who goes on to give generalized advice from what seems like her own predetermined agenda.

A further example of nurses' failure to acknowledge the experience and knowledge a patient brings to the encounter, and to offer advice accordingly, is exemplified by the extract below from a taped admission:

Nurse 3 (3):   *Brilliant. The operation will take about an hour and then you'll be going to theatre for another hour, so you'll be off the ward for a good couple of hours. So tell them to leave it for a good few hours before they phone up, probably very early afternoon, say one o'clock-ish to see how you are. When you come back you will have a drip up, just to keep you hydrated until you're drinking on Thursday morning. Um . . . that's basically all you'll have. We'll come to you every hour when you come back to the ward, make sure you're comfortable and not in any pain, even if it's a bit of discomfort, tell us and we can give you an injection to take it away, and also put in your anti-sickness injections in with that, 'cause of the anaesthetic'. It depends how you react to anaesthetics. How have you been with the other ones?*

Patient: *Alright.*
Nurse 3 (3):   *You've been alright. The chances are that you'll be fine then.*
Patient: *I just sleep like a log.*

Thus, although information-giving was evident in the recorded interactions, the process often did not exhibit the characteristics of an empowering approach in that it was not collaborative or participatory and is unlikely to have resulted in patient empowerment. Other potential opportunities for collaborating with patients were also missed by nurses on this ward. For example, observation and field notes contained numerous instances of nurses updating care plans at the foot of the bed without consulting the patient.

On Ward 2 a different picture of practice emerged. Data analysis indicated that nurses were engaged in certain health education activities, and that these and other interactions were characterized by the health-promoting principles described above. Observation and field notes contained many examples of information and explanations being offered to patients, and this appeared to be integrated into care and given in response to need. For example, as the ward round moved on from a patient's bed area, a nurse was observed explaining the medical team's diagnosis in response to the patient's comment that he had not understood all of it. Other examples of education about patients' diagnoses and their medication were also recorded. Analysis of the recorded interactions and field notes revealed that nurses used a collaborative, individualized and empowering approach. The following extract from a recording of a nurse–patient interaction about medication illustrates a more collaborative approach which acknowledges the patient's existing knowledge:

Nurse 11(2):   *So when would you take this, do you think?*
Patient: *Well if I ever get that pain there. But some days I only get it once a day or not at all. I don't take it if I've got no pain.*
Nurse 11(2):   *That's right. And do you have a rest at the same time?*
Patient: *Yes, I always sit down for about 10 minutes, quarter of an hour after I usually get that pain if I've done a bit of hoovering, you know.*
Nurse 11(2):   *That's right. And you were saying yesterday that you know how much you can do and when you've got to stop.*

During the bedside handovers which were observed and/or audio-recorded it was noted that patients were as fully involved as possible, and were asked to describe their morning or afternoon for the oncoming nurse. An example of a typical handover interaction is given below:

Nurse 15 (2):   *I'm X and I'm going to be looking after you this afternoon.*
Patient: *OK.*
Nurse 15 (2):   *Alright, I know that you've seen me but I haven't been looking after you for too long.*
Patient: *No, no, I've seen you around.*
Nurse 5 (2):(to patient) *Do you want to tell X what has been happening this morning?*

Patient:	*Well, yes. I mean I had a couple of X-rays and a couple of scans.*
Nurse 15 (2):	*Oh, good.*
Patient:	*Um. . . I was going to have one, but when I told the young doctor about the swelling in my ankles and when I saw the consultant they had the X-rays, so he said, 'Are you alright?' and I said 'Yes' and he said, 'You don't sound it' and I said 'Look at this' you know.*
Nurse 15 (2):	*Is that a new problem then, or just happened?*
Patient:	*I don't have it very often, but I told the nurse about it.*
Nurse 15 (2):	*Don't worry, it's not an unusual problem.*

(Tape-recorded handover)

Similarly, care plans were updated with the patients and had notices attached indicating that the permission of the patient should be sought prior to reading them.

Thus overall it appeared that the nurses' practice on this ward more closely approximated to a health-promoting approach to their interactions than that of the nurses on Wards 1 and 3. Analysis of the perceived influences on practice and cross-case comparison between wards illuminates possible reasons for this differential development.

Influences on practice

On Wards 1 and 3, the general approach to care which was observed appeared to be based on a philosophy of care which was not consistent with the development of an empowering approach to health education or health–nursing interactions by nurses on the ward. Field notes, non-participant observation notes and recorded interactions all indicated that the nurses were operating predominantly with what appeared to be a medical model philosophy of care, with its focus on the patient as a collection of symptoms of physical illness, and a traditional distinction between professional and lay competence and knowledge. This is apparent both from the data presented above and from the researcher's field notes about other observations that nurses were orientated to completing tasks. The following comment from the researcher's field notes illustrates this:

> The staff tend to be a bit orientated to getting the work done: I have heard them mention in passing that they have 'already done their observations' or their patient dependency scores.

(Ward 3)

Clearly this philosophy militates against the incorporation of a health focus and a collaborative, holistic and individualized approach to care.

Related to this was the way in which Wards 1 and 3 were managed and the allocation or organization of nursing care as evidenced at the end of shift handovers. The ward sisters had a clearly defined hierarchical management style such that individual staff members had little decision-making power or autonomy in their work. They were allocated work by the ward sister or person in charge at the beginning of a shift, and their allocated patients changed frequently, often on a daily basis, resulting in a lack of continuity of care and individual responsibility for patients. The ward sisters were also observed to carry out the drug and ward rounds and to make decisions about patient care which overrode the individual nurse caring for a particular patient, thus appearing to result in a lack of autonomy for individual practitioners.

The lack of continuity and responsibility for individual patients' care appeared to prevent individualized and holistic health education or health–nursing interactions based on a therapeutic nurse–patient relationship. Thus this system of organizing nursing care appeared to derive from and reinforce the predominant ideology of patients being seen as a series of physical care tasks, and thus the empowering of patients through health education or health-promoting nursing was excluded from the nurses' agendas.

The data collected also indicated that a lack of knowledge and skills relevant to health education and health promotion may have contributed to its absence from practice on Wards 1 and 3. Several nurses mentioned this to the researcher in informal conversation, and this is verified by some of the examples of information-giving recorded as outlined earlier. Most nurses on Wards 1 and 3 had trained with a traditional curriculum, as opposed to a Project 2000 (United Kingdom Central Council for Nurses, Midwives and Health Visitors, 1986) curriculum, and they reported informally to the researcher that they had received little post-registration education and/or input on health education and promotion principles and skills. This perceived deficiency was confirmed in the analysis of questionnaires completed by nurses on these wards (see Macleod Clark *et al.*, 1992). Responses indicated that only five of the 17 qualified nurses who completed questionnaires (Ward 1, $n = 10$; Ward 3, $n = 7$) had undertaken post-registration courses which may have helped them to gain knowledge and skills relevant to their health education role. Of these 5 nurses, three had completed the ENB 998 Teaching and Assessing course, one had a Certificate in Education and one had undertaken an RSA counselling course. Therefore, whilst these courses may have been indirectly beneficial, none of the nurses had taken post-registration courses aimed specifically at enhancing their health education and health promotion knowledge and skills. Responses to a further questionnaire item revealed that the nurses were aware of the need for development of this nature to enhance their role. When asked whether they needed further education or training with regard to health education and health promotion, 8 nurses ($n = 10$) of those on Ward 1 and 5 nurses ($n = 6$) of those on Ward 2 replied 'Yes'. One nurse's written comment aptly indicated the less than adequate preparation and the desire for further education. She wrote:

> As a student our preparation for health educators was very limited as the curriculum was aimed at illness and not health. I feel that some formal education in health promotion would be extremely beneficial . . .

Clearly then, such limitations in the nurses' knowledge and skills are likely to have prevented the development of their role, and this helps to explain the form of current practice presented above.

In contrast, particular influences on practice were identified on Ward 2 which may have facilitated the development of the nurses' health promotion role towards patients. The ward philosophy appeared to be a key influential factor in the development of the collaborative health education and health–nursing interactions seen on the ward. Central elements of the philosophy underpinning care on Ward 2 appeared to be a respect for patients and their rights, as well as individualized, holistic care, partnership, patient control and continuity of the nurse–patient relationship. These features were written into the ward philosophy document, and clearly they are congruent with health nursing and an empowerment approach to health education. These characteristics also equate with what has been described as the New Nursing philosophy (Beardshaw and Robinson, 1990; Salvage, 1990). The philosophy was also made accessible to patients by having available an album of ward photographs for patients to look at and read through. These illustrated valued principles, such as partnership, 'in action'. This not only indicates that the philosophy was actively being shared in practice, but that it forms a further example of the collaborative approach taken by the nurses towards the patients on Ward 2. Several of the nurses commented on the importance of the ward philosophy when asked in a reflective interview to identify the reasons why they felt that health education had developed on the ward. One suggested:

> I mean, people have a right to sort of know what's going on with their health, and to make their decisions for themselves. And I think it's just a thing that's evolved on the ward . . . it's very much sort of part of the ward philosophy . . . that everyone believes in.
>
> (Taped interview)

A second influence perceived by both the nurses and the researcher as being beneficial to the development of health education concerned the democratic manner in which the ward was run. This was closely associated with the well-established system of Primary Nursing in operation on the ward. Beardshaw and Robinson (1990) define Primary Nursing as the allocation of 24-hour responsibility for each patient's care to a trained primary nurse who acts with the active collaboration of the patient. It also requires devolved decision-making and the absence of a nursing hierarchy on the ward, both of which were clearly evident on Ward 2. This was perceived as favourable by several of the nurses. One commented:

> When X (ward sister) started here, and she came with the idea of introducing Primary Nursing . . . um, as a way of giving us more control . . . in our practice and a way of giving us more power, and I think it's just evolved in that we want to now give our patients more power as well.
>
> (Taped interview)

The researcher's field notes also document examples of the lack of hierarchy – individual nurses planned and implemented care for their patients without directives from the ward sister. In addition, any enquiries about individual patients from relatives or other health care professionals were redirected by the ward sister or co-ordinating nurse to the primary nurse caring for that particular patient. That is, the ward sister or co-ordinating nurse did not erode the autonomy of other primary nurses by assuming responsibility for communicating about their patients.

A further potential influence that was identified concerned the general educational or knowledge level of the staff. Data collected via questionnaire (see Macleod Clark *et al.*, 1992) indicated that this was relatively high compared to the other two case study wards. Six respondents or 43% ($n = 14$) currently held or were undertaking the Bachelor of Nursing degree, two (14%) had diplomas and three (21%) had completed ENB approved courses. In addition, the ward sister was highly qualified, holding both a Diploma and a Masters Degree in Nursing, as well as a Certificate in Further Education. In contrast, the ward sisters on Wards 1 and 3 had not studied beyond the academic level of their original nursing qualification. The nurses on Ward 2 also had structured time and opportunities to share knowledge gained following study days, and many were also student mentors, which may have given the staff an incentive to increase their own knowledge base.

The researcher also noted that there seemed to be a sense of social cohesion between all members of the staff on Ward 2, with nurses taking time out together on the ward to develop teamworking skills, as well as socializing outside working hours.

To summarize, a number of potential influences on practice were identified which served either to constrain or to facilitate nurses' health promotion practice on Wards 1 and 3 and Ward 2, respectively. These concerned the philosophy of care underpinning practice and the associated organization of care, as well as the nurses' education levels. It is suggested below that an explanation for their influence on nurses' health promotion practice lies in considering the extent to which these features offer a framework for nurse empowerment.

Discussion

Philosophy and organization of care as a route to nurse empowerment

It is clear from what has been written about the New Nursing approach to care, which was evident on Ward 2, that this has the potential to empower nurses. Salvage (1990) traces the origins of the New Nursing in the UK back to the early 1970s, and links its inception to developments such as the women's movement, which began to challenge nursing's subordination to medicine, and nascent consumerism, which provoked a re-evaluation of the client–expert relationship. Key texts (Chapman, 1985; Wright, 1985; Pearson, 1988) identify the practitioner and the clinical base as central to the New Nursing, in contrast to previous bureaucratic and task-oriented approaches. Beardshaw and Robinson (1990) suggest that the new approach is based on a highly skilled nurse practitioner who will have the competence and confidence to give individualized care. They contrast New Nursing to past and present systems in which competence is based on ability to undertake a variety of tasks and 'get by and cope'. Making nurses' skills, competence and confidence central to good quality care is clearly more likely to engender their autonomy and empowerment than the latter approach described by Beardshaw and Robinson, which was in evidence on Wards 1 and 3.

The New Nursing is also associated with changes in the division of labour and organization of care on the ward, represented by Primary Nursing. That is, Primary Nursing forms a vehicle for operationalizing this particular approach to care. Advocates of this system of organizing patient care have highlighted the fact that its ability to achieve its objectives is crucially dependent on the autonomy or empowerment of individual nurse practitioners. Manthey (1992) states that Primary Nursing recognizes the value of individuals at all levels, puts them in control of their own actions, and facilitates a very high level of quality by enabling and empowering nurses to perform at their maximum capacity. Pearson (1988) outlines the relationship between New Nursing principles and Primary Nursing, proposing that individualization of care means, in effect, autonomy for the patient, but this cannot happen if the direct care-giver who is with the patient is powerless to allow him to act on the decisions he makes. Pearson concludes, therefore, that autonomy for the nurse is necessary to allow autonomy for the patient. Consequently, the management structure associated with Primary Nursing focuses on the primary nurse, unlike conventional settings where the hierarchy moves power upwards and away from the practitioner (Salvage, 1990). Pearson believes that the lack of autonomy inherent in traditional hierarchical structures not only impairs the quality of care, but also reduces the patient's power by reducing the autonomy needed for the nurse to develop partnership with the patient. This theoretical relationship between lack of nurse autonomy and the inability to promote autonomy in patients was clearly seen in practice on both Wards 1 and 3, where traditional hierarchical systems of ward management were in operation. In contrast, Primary Nursing is associated with a flattened ward hierarchy with responsibility for decision-making devolved to individual primary nurses and the ward sister acting as an adviser or co-ordinator as opposed to a supervisor. Again, these features were evident from the data collected on case study Ward 2.

The principle of autonomous primary nurses can be linked to the calls in the health promotion literature (e.g. Clarke, 1991; Tones, 1993) that nurses themselves must first be empowered in order for them to be able to empower others as part of the new approach to health education. However, to date there has been a lack of empirical evidence exploring the link between this approach to care organization and management and the development of nurses' health-promoting practice at ward level.

Whilst not directly exploring health promotion, the findings from McMahon's (1990) study on Primary Nursing shed some light on this area and also bear a similarities to the findings of this study. McMahon's description of the relationships on the hierarchical wards bears a close similarity to the findings from the observational data from Wards 1 and 3 in the present study. For example, he states that on one ward, the ward sister seemed to control the working patterns of all her nurses, and the nurses were allocated to different 'ends' of the ward for each shift, and therefore did not necessarily look after the same patients on consecutive shifts. Conversely, on the Primary Nursing ward the nurse in charge of the shift appeared not to wield the potential power gained from that position, but rather allowed the other nurses to work autonomously. Examples of the ways in which this was manifested are again similar to the findings from Ward 2 in this study. For instance, McMahon found that enquiries about patients were redirected by the co-ordinating nurse to the individual nurse who was looking after that particular patient. This was also observed to be the case when doctors, other health care professionals and relatives enquired about patients on Ward 2 in this study.

McMahon concludes that, on the wards with a hierarchical management structure, power seemed to rest in the position at the top of the hierarchy, with that person directing the actions of her peers and checking that they were completed satisfactorily. On the Primary Nursing wards, power was vested in individuals – nurses sought less approval for their actions, rarely asked for guidance and generally acted more autonomously than on the traditionally managed wards. McMahon recommends that further research confirming these findings would be of value, as would an investigation to determine whether these differences have a positive influence on the quality of patient care. The findings derived from the case study wards in this study appear to be congruent with those of McMahon. These findings also suggest that one way in which lateral management may positively influence the quality of care is through its association with more individualized and participatory health-promoting interactions with patients. (It should be noted, however, that patients' perceptions regarding the quality improvement of these types of interactions were not elicited, and critics such as Salvage (1992) draw on sociological literature to suggest that patients' preferences for partnership, as opposed to hierarchy, may not be straight-forward.)

It is proposed that the mechanism whereby this management style facilitates health-promoting interactions may be explained by the mediating influence of the nurses' own empowerment. This hypothesis is explored more fully below, following an analysis of the contribution that nurses' educational preparation may make to their experience of empowerment.

The potential contribution of education to nurse empowerment

The findings from the case study wards also revealed that there was a marked difference in the educational attainment of nurses on Ward 2, compared to those on Wards 1 and 3. This may also be related to the nurses' ability to engage in health-promoting interactions with patients, via the mediating mechanism of increasing the nurses' sense of empowerment. The content of the education experience may be important in fostering this. Tones (1993) suggests that the proper development of nurses' health promotion role has obvious implications for training and the nursing curriculum. He maintains that the suggestion should be considered that assertiveness training should form an important part of the repertoire of social and education skills which will support the nurse's health promotion function. Clarke (1991) develops a similar argument, advocating the inclusion of communication skills, personal effectiveness, counselling, assertiveness training and self-exploration as examples of the means whereby nurses, through education, may have the opportunity to begin to develop an awareness of 'self' and to build the self-confidence which goes along with it. She maintains that nurses' preparation for a health education role must include learning about 'self', if giving up a controlling role and being 'real' to patients is to be a core feature of their health education practice. Clearly, exposure to these areas is likely to have an empowering effect on nurses. If they are equipped through education with a range of personal and social skills, they are perhaps more likely to feel in control of the practice situations in which they find themselves. Such situations include both encounters between professionals (e.g. nurse and doctor) and those between nurses and patients. The thesis of this chapter is that the corollary of increasing nurses' sense of control or empowerment is that they are then less likely to take control of interactions with patients.

In addition, the processes involved in the educational experience have the potential to contribute to empowering those who are learning. With reference to trainee health educators, D'Onofrio (1992) and Williams (1995) argue that the experiences to which they are exposed need to be empowering and participative, rather than prescriptive. Fahlberg *et al.* (1991) also recommend this, and suggest that professionals will disempower their clients if they adopt authoritarian approaches. They argue that the latter lead to professionals' need to retain control over service users in order to meet their own ego needs. The implication is that nurse educators need to be cognizant of both the content and the processes involved in pre- and post-registration education programmes in order to foster nurse empowerment.

Characteristics of empowerment, and their relationship to health promotion in nursing practice

The findings from this study suggest that exposure to further education as well as certain features of the philosophy, organization and management of care may have an empowering effect on nurses, and that this is linked to their ability to empower patients as part of their health promotion role. A closer analysis of the concept of empowerment offers a framework for understanding the relationship between nurses' empowerment and their ability to foster it with patients or clients.

According to Keiffer (1984), empowerment is associated with such characteristics as mutual support, support systems, personal efficacy, competence, self-sufficiency and self-esteem. The findings from this study indicate that many of these applied to the nurses on Ward 2 (see Figure 1.1). These nurses appeared to enjoy support both from their colleagues and from the ward sister. This may have been, in part, a function of the Primary Nursing system in operation, which was conducive to the development of teamworking skills. This was in contrast to the situation in Ward 1 in particular, where it was found that nurses were not supported or valued in their work. The competence element of empowerment described by Keiffer was also in evidence on Ward 2. That is, the New Nursing philosophy helped to ensure that nurses' competence was valued, rather than their ability to complete tasks. The nurses' sense of competence may also have been enhanced by their comparatively high levels of educational attainment.

The idea that personal efficacy, self-sufficiency and self-esteem are associated with empowerment is also postulated by Tones (1991). These concepts, too, can be applied to the case study ward findings. Tones draws on the theoretical literature pertaining to the concept of control in order to explain this relationship. He outlines Lewis' (1986, personal communication) typology of control, including the idea of processual control, which is relevant here. This notion of control concerns the extent to which an individual might be involved in discussions or decisions affecting any given event or situation, and is related to beliefs about control (Tones, 1991). Beliefs about control are considered to be valuable and to contribute to self-efficacy and thus to empowerment. This notion of processual control can be applied to the findings from Ward 2, where the methods of work organization were found to be characterized by the devolved decision-making which is a hallmark of Primary Nursing. That is, the fact that individual nurses were able to make decisions about patient care and to participate in decisions affecting ward functioning afforded them feelings of control, thus contributing to their own sense of empowerment. Once again, the contrast with the findings from Wards 1 and 3 in this respect is striking, in that on the latter wards individual nurses appeared to lack any sense of control. Instead, consistent with the task orientation of these wards, the ward sister assumed responsibility for decision-making.

In his consideration of the relationship between control and empowerment, Tones (1991) cites Phares' assertion that individuals who feel they have control of their situation are likely to exhibit behaviour that will better enable them to cope with potentially threatening situations than individuals who feel that chance or other non-controllable factors will determine whether their

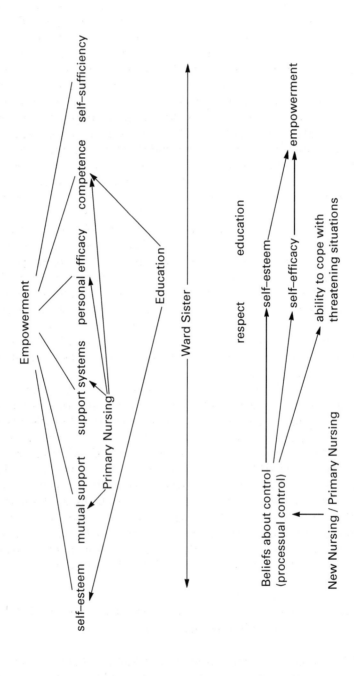

Figure 1.1 The relationship between features of Ward 2 and components of empowerment; adapted from Keiffer (1984) and Tones (1991)

behaviour will be successful. In essence, then, coping behaviour in a health-threatening situation is believed to be related to perceived degree of control. Applying this idea to a different context – the nurses on the case study wards – may also be of relevance. It is possible that an empowering, health-promoting nurse–patient interaction which requires the nurse to relinquish her role as 'expert' and acknowledge the patient's power represents a potentially threatening situation for the nurse. If, as Phares argues, the ability to cope with this threatening situation is related to the degree of control possessed, then this may explain why the nurses on Ward 2 were better able to acknowledge the patients' perspective, as was evidenced, for example, during bedside handovers. That is, it is possible that this was because they experienced a greater degree of control than their counterparts on Wards 1 and 3. Thus the degree of control offered to individual nurses as a function of the philosophy, organization and management of care on the ward may contribute to their empowerment and help to explain the differential development of health promotion practice observed on the case study wards.

The contribution that self-esteem may make to empowerment is commented on by Keiffer (1984), and Tones (1991) also suggests that there is an interaction between control and self-esteem. The greater degree of control enjoyed by the nurses on Ward 2 may also have been influential in enhancing their self-esteem. However, as Tones points out, many other factors influence self-esteem, such as being treated with respect by significant others. Nurses on Ward 2 were observed to be treated with respect both by colleagues and by the ward sister and this, together with their level of educational attainment and autonomy in their work, may have fostered their self-esteem and thus their empowerment.

In contrast, this was not found to apply to the nurses on Wards 1 and 3. In essence, Gibson's (1991) description of the characteristics that define an absence of empowerment – powerlessness, subordination, paternalism and a loss of a sense of control – are all relevant to the situation in which nurses on these wards found themselves working. The lack of evidence of any empowering interactions with patients may have been due, as suggested by Fahlberg *et al.* (1991) to the nurses' need to retain control over them in order to meet their own ego needs. Alternatively, applying Phares' analysis (cited by Tones, 1991), this finding could be explained by the nurses being unable to cope with the potentially threatening prospect of patients assuming a greater degree of control within interactions, due to their own inner feelings of lack of control over their work situation and decision-making.

Empowerment of nurses – a key to their social and political role in health promotion?

Thus far, this chapter has been concerned with the health education component of the hospital nurse's role, i.e. that part which is enacted at the level of the one-to-one encounter with patients or clients and carers. To conclude the case for advocating the empowerment of hospital-based nurses, it is pertinent at this point to turn to nurses' broader role in the structural, as opposed to individual, component of health promotion.

The need for nurses to take on a more political role in order to promote health has been recognized and advocated by a number of different commentators (Coxon, 1986; Maglacas, 1988; Williams, 1989; Butterfield, 1990; Watts, 1990; Delaney, 1991). Congruent with the findings of this study, it has also been suggested that nurses' focus has traditionally been on the individual, without recognition of the social context of behaviour and their responsibilities to facilitate change at this level. For example, Butterfield (1990) asserts that nurses pay more attention to individual attitudes and symptoms of poor health than to its socio-economic causes, and that viewing the world from such a perspective does not allow the possibility of working to alter the system itself or empowering clients to do so. Maglacas (1988) also argues that nurses' health promotion potential is far from being realized, and she ascribes this in part to nurses' lack of understanding of and involvement in the social, economic and political realm.

These assertions about nurses' lack of engagement in the broader field of health promotion, as opposed to health education, are substantiated by the findings from this study. That is, data from the case study wards revealed little evidence of nurses lobbying, networking or working collaboratively with others in order to influence policies and environments in the interests of health. Rather, their health promotion contribution, if it had developed, appeared to be focused on individual patients/clients and carers. In order to provide a possible explanation for this, and thus to consider the implications for nursing practice, the research of Williams (1987, 1989) and Gott and O'Brien (1990) is relevant here. They claim that, in order to develop a leading role in health promotion, the nursing profession needs to free itself from subordination and increase its autonomy and self-determination. Williams asserts that the socio-historical situation of nursing, past and present, is one of subordination and limited power based on interactions between social hierarchies of class and gender. This condition, she argues, has consciousness-structuring effects that explain the profession's preoccupation with what she refers to as 'atomistic' health promotion, derived from the medical model. Williams maintains that the structural and ideological conditions that subordinate the nursing profession are the same as those that result in an inequitable distribution of health and which render an atomistic model of health promotion inappropriate and ineffective. Gott and O'Brien draw a similar conclusion. They suggest that the nursing profession has a near universal subordinate status *vis-à-vis* other professions and interests, and that its agenda is divided between the demands of its employing organizations and the priorities of its superordinate allied professions. They suggest that nurses are afforded little authority or control within the health care system, and that this directly contradicts the ethos and ethics of health promotion which attempts to address inequities and promote meaningful participation in programmes of health.

In essence, the suggestion is that if nurses are to be able to develop a broader and more political role at the level of health promotion, then empowerment of the profession or empowerment at what could be considered to be a macro level needs to occur. Reference to Tones' (1991) description of the process of empowerment of groups of individuals highlights a way in which this may be achieved, and has some relevance to the findings of this study. He suggests that healthy public policy is needed to remedy health-damaging inequalities and to create an empowered populace. Paradoxically, however, the most significant way to change existing policy is through substantial popular pressure. He argues that, in order to create such pressure, people need to believe they can influence the course of events and have the skills to do so – that is, they need to be empowered. Essentially, the reasoning here is that one way of effecting change in policies and the social infrastructure is through the empowerment of individuals. Whilst Tones' description refers to empowerment for health promotion changes, these ideas could also be applied to the position of the nursing profession within society. That is, equality and autonomy for the profession at a social or macro level, as advocated by Williams (1987, 1989) and Gott and O'Brien (1990), may be achieved through the empowerment of its individual members. It is possible to suggest that one precursor of this individual empowerment is the shift to a philosophy of care which facilitates this. That is, if the philosophy of care and the resultant autonomy and control enjoyed by the nurses on Ward 2 were to become a more widespread phenomenon in hospital ward settings, this might eventually culminate in self-determination for the profession via the empowerment it would offer individual practitioners. In turn, this empowerment or self-determination of the profession could facilitate a more comprehensive development of nurses' health-promoting potential by allowing engagement in broader policy and political activities.

Further insights into this relationship are offered by a consideration of Keiffer's (1984) conceptualization of empowerment as a developmental sequence or a process of becoming. He outlines four stages, the first of which is characterized by the participation of the individual as exploratory, unknown and unsure, while authority and power structures are demystified. The deliberate dismantling of the hierarchical/ bureaucratic management structure was an organizational feature of both Ward 2 and the hospital in which it was situated (Fox, 1993), and is relevant to this stage of empowerment. The second stage is termed the 'era of advancement', and is characterized by a mentoring relationship as well as supportive peer relationships. There are opportunities for collaboration and mutually supportive problem-solving, and the individual develops mechanisms for action and accepts responsibility for choices. Keiffer also suggests that rudimentary political skills are developed at this stage. This second stage in the process of empowerment parallels many of the characteristics of the nurses' work situation on Ward 2, although the data indicated that they may not yet have begun to develop political skills in relation to health promotion.

Keiffer's third stage highlights how the philosophy of nursing on Ward 2 may contribute to changes in the status and autonomy of the profession as a whole. He describes this as an 'era of incorporation', in which activities are focused on confronting and contending with the permanence and painfulness of structural or institutional barriers to self-determination. Thus in the context of the current discussion, this may involve confronting some of the barriers to developing a health promotion role referred to by Williams (1987, 1989) and Gott and O'Brien (1990). Keiffer states that this phase is further characterized by the development of organizational, leadership and survival skills. The fourth stage is the 'era of commitment', in which the individual integrates new personal knowledge and skills into the reality of everyday life.

If it were to become a more widespread phenomenon, it is possible that the ward-based empowerment of hospital nurses observed in this study would have the potential to evolve into a process which leads to changes in the status and autonomy of the nursing profession more generally, as advocated by Williams (1987) and Gott and O'Brien (1990). Combined with appropriate health promotion knowledge and skills and changes in the organization of hospital nurses' work, this could then facilitate not only individual health education with patients, but also the development of nurses' broader health promotion role.

Whilst Keiffer's sequential stages offer a potential framework for conceptualizing how nursing may move forward to embrace a broader health promotion role, it should be noted that there was a lack of evidence to suggest that the nurses on Ward 2 had reached the third and fourth stages of this process of becoming empowered. It is likely that considerable barriers to achieving this could be encountered. These, and other challenges to operationalizing the concept of empowerment in acute care settings are outlined below.

Empowering nurses – the challenges

This chapter has presented evidence which suggests that there is a relationship between nurses' own sense of empowerment and their ability to foster it in patients as part of their health promotion role. The data collected from three contrasting case study wards indicates that the philosophy upon which nursing care is based, the system by which care is organized and delivered and the educational qualifications of nurses may be instrumental in creating or diminishing nurses' experience of empowerment. Whilst the importance of nurse empowerment is argued for here, it is also likely that a number of challenges will need to be faced, both in achieving elsewhere the level of democracy and autonomy of the nurses on Ward 2, and in moving beyond this to an emancipated nursing profession that is able to contribute its full health promotion potential.

The answer to the first of these challenges perhaps lies in the ability to implement and sustain a system of organizing care such as Primary Nursing, in which nurses are autonomous and accountable practitioners. Manthey (1992) stresses that the extent to which Primary Nursing can become a widespread phenomenon is crucially dependent on the organizational theory on which the administrative structure is founded, and the attitude of management towards it. Hospitals are historically highly bureaucratic and hierarchical organizations, and the switch to decentralized decision-making and a flattened hierarchy may prove difficult, both ideologically and practically. In addition, Primary Nursing requires proficient, qualified nurses to deliver care and to assume 24-hour responsibility for this, rather than qualified nurses taking on a more administrative ward 'manager' role with care delivery delegated to less highly qualified staff. This, too, may be hard to sustain from a resource point of view. Difficulties in recruiting and retaining sufficient qualified nurses, as well as budget restrictions, have led to skill mix reviews and staffing levels which are far from conducive to the system of organizing and delivering care advocated here. There is a need to balance historical traditions and real resource issues with the creation of opportunities wherever possible for nurses and patients to derive benefits from skilled and empowered nurses delivering care at the bedside. That is, in the context of current health care reforms, managers and policy-makers should strive for democratic decision-making, a culture which values nurses' competence and skills, in which autonomy and independent decision-making are encouraged and nurses experience peer and managerial support. Evaluation of clinical outcomes where these characteristics are *in situ* would seem to be essential in order to make a case for skilled nursing care delivery.

Even where the values of New Nursing are upheld and operationalized through Primary Nursing, challenges to the goal of empowering nurses remain. Whilst this chapter has focused on empowerment as a consequence of nursing philosophy, organization of care delivery and nurse education, a consideration of the broader context of the nursing profession's position in society and its relationship to medicine has also been referred to. The challenge to nurse empowerment posed by the traditional place of nursing as unskilled and unpaid women's work, and its long history of suppression and subordination to medicine, is considerable. In her sociological critique of the New Nursing, Salvage (1992) makes this point. She suggests that in order to work in a therapeutic partnership with patients, major changes to both the occupational socialization of nurses and the organization of hospital work are needed. She reminds us that 'The division of health care labour, from doctors to care assistants, still rests on traditional inequalities in gender, race and education, so tinkering with its internal boundaries [through the implementation of New Nursing] will make little difference without broader social change' (Salvage, 1992).

The empowerment of nurses cannot be divorced from the wider social context in which nursing takes place, and changes to fundamental and deep-rooted inequalities are likely to be slow. Such inequalities are perhaps epitomized nowhere more clearly than in the hierarchical and patriarchal hospital setting in which the dominance of medicine and the medical model has been paramount. The closure of Nursing Development Units (NDUs) in which New Nursing and Primary Nursing were pioneered (see Salvage, 1992) is testimony to the difficulties encountered in challenging orthodoxy and the creation of autonomous nurses. Nevertheless, other NDUs and nursing beds survive. In addition, the thesis presented above is that increasing nurses' sense of empowerment at the ward level may culminate in greater autonomy for the profession as a whole. The recent changes in nurse education – its move into higher education, the education of students about the socio-historical and political position of nurses, as well as an emphasis on reflection – are also likely to result in a professional group that is more informed and autonomous than previous generations of nurses. Recent changes in the scope of nursing practice and the establishment of 'Nurse Practitioners' in primary and secondary care may also offer opportunities for empowering nurses. If the inherent danger of creating 'mini-doctors' from these posts is avoided, they have the potential to offer increased autonomy, independent decision-making and enhanced control for nurses, whilst at the same time helping to break down the traditional hierarchy between nurses' and doctors' work.

A further challenge resides not so much in the obstacles to achieving nurse empowerment, but in the likely consequences of it. That is, there are risks involved for those who are sufficiently empowered to speak up and challenge vested political and economic interests as part of a broader health promotion role. At the organizational or Trust level, whistleblowing is discouraged and may incur penalties, and the politicization of nurses on a broader scale is inevitably difficult in view of their position as employees of the State.

A final point worthy of consideration concerns not so much the challenge of empowering nurses, but the issue of empowering patients in acute care settings. Facilitating the ability of patients to exert greater control over their care and decision-making while they are in hospital may not always be appropriate or desirable, and there is a danger that patient empowerment and participation could be applied *carte blanche* as an inherently 'good thing'. Current opinion and research suggest that discretion and selective application of theory in practice are required. Salvage (1992), for example, draws on Parsons' (1951) classic thesis on the sick role to illustrate the inherent dangers of neglecting the therapeutic potential of a hierarchical relationship between professional and patient. She suggests that the part played by faith or belief during illness may make a hierarchical relationship beneficial, and that demystifying it may be disadvantageous. Further research is needed on the reality of patient preferences while in hospital, but some evidence exists (see, for example, Waterworth and Luker, 1990) to suggest that patients may not always choose a participative approach to their care and treatment. None the less, the solution does not lie in a universal return to professional domination and hierarchical relationships which exclude patient participation and control. The challenge for nurses rests in sound application of their assessment and communication skills in order that they are able to monitor continuously patient preferences for degrees of control and dependency. These preferences are likely to vary both between individuals and within a particular individual during the period of his or her admission to the acute care setting.

Such challenges may be difficult to overcome, but the findings from this study bear witness to the possibility of empowering hospital-based nurses, and indicate that this may yield improvements in the quality of care by enhancing the quality of their interactions with patients/clients such that they are more consistent with empowering, health-promoting nursing.

Endnote

1.1 The author would like to acknowledge that the study described here formed part of a larger research project funded by the Department of Health (Macleod Clark *et al.*, 1992). The views expressed are those of the author and are not intended to represent those of the Department of Health.

References

Beardshaw,V. and Robinson, R. 1990: *New for old? Prospects for nursing in the 1990s.* Research Report No. 8. London: King's Fund Institute.

Benson, A. 1991: *Empowerment: from rhetoric to reality.* Unpublished BEd Thesis, South Bank University, London.

Butterfield, P.G. 1990: Thinking upstream: nurturing a conceptual understanding of the societal context of health behaviour. *Advances in Nursing Science* **12**, 1–8.

Carlson-Catalano, J. 1992: Empowering nurses for professional practice. *Nursing Outlook* **40**, 139–42.

Chapman, C. 1985: *Theory of nursing: practical application.* London: Harper and Row.

Clarke, A.C. 1991: Nurses as role models and health educators. *Journal of Advanced Nursing* **16**, 1178–84.

Clay, T. 1992: Education and empowerment: securing nurses' future. *International Nursing Review* **39**, 15–18.

Coxon, J. 1986: Health education: a learning dilemma. *Senior Nurse* **15**, 22–4.

Cribb, A. and Dines, A. 1993: What is health promotion? In Dines, A. and Cribb, A. (eds), *Health promotion: concepts and practice.* Oxford: Blackwell Scientific Publications, 20–32.

Dalton, C. 1990: The sleeping giant awakes. *The Canadian Nurse* **89**, 16–18.

Delaney, F. 1991: Getting the message across. *Nursing* **4**, 24–5.

Department of Health 1989: *A strategy for nursing.* London: HMSO.

Department of Health 1993: *Vision for the future: the nursing, midwifery and health visiting contribution to health and health care*. London: HMSO.

D'Onofrio, C. N. 1992: Theory and empowerment of health education practitioners. *Health Education Quarterly* **19**, 385–403.

Downie, R.S., Fyfe, C. and Tannahill, A. 1990: *Health promotion: models and values* (revised reprint). Oxford: Oxford Medical Publications.

Duffy, M.E. 1987: Methodological triangulation: a vehicle for quantitative and qualitative research methods. *Image* **19**, 130–3.

Fahlberg, L.L., Poulin, A.L., Girdano, D.A. and Dusek, D.E. 1991: Empowerment as an emerging approach to health education. *Journal of the Institute of Health Education* **22**, 185–93.

Field, P.A. and Morse, J.M. 1992: *Nursing research: the application of qualitative approaches*. London: Chapman and Hall.

Fox, P. 1993: *New roles within a new culture*. Paper presented at the International Council of Nurses Conference, 20–25 June 1993, Madrid.

Freire, P. 1968: *Pedagogy of the oppressed*. New York: Seabury Press.

Gibson, C. 1991: A concept analysis of empowerment. *Journal of Advanced Nursing* **16**, 354–61.

Gott, M. and O'Brien, M. 1990: *The role of the nurse in health promotion: policies, perspectives and practice*. Unpublished report of a two-year research project funded by the Department of Health. Milton Keynes: Department of Health and Social Welfare, The Open University.

Johnston, I. 1988: *A study of the promotion of healthy lifestyles by hospital-based staff*. Unpublished MSc Thesis, University of Birmingham, Birmingham.

Keiffer, C. 1984: Citizen empowerment: a developmental perspective. *Prevention in Human Services* **3**, 9–36.

Kendall, S. 1991: *An analysis of the health visitor–client interaction: the influence of the health visiting process on client participation*. Unpublished PhD Thesis, King's College, University of London, London.

Lask, S. 1987: Beliefs and behaviour in health education. *Nursing* **3**, 681–3.

Latter, S. 1994: *Health education and health promotion: perceptions and practices of nurses in acute care settings*. Unpublished PhD Thesis, King's College, University of London, London.

Macdonald, G. and Bunton, R. 1992: Health promotion: discipline or disciplines? In Bunton, R. and Macdonald, G. (eds), *Health promotion: disciplines and diversity*. London: Routledge, 6–19.

Macleod Clark, J. 1993: From sick nursing to health nursing: evolution or revolution. In Wilson-Barnett, J. and Macleod Clark, J. (eds), *Research in health promotion and nursing*. Basingstoke: Macmillan, 256–70.

Macleod Clark, J. Haverty, S. and Kendall, S. 1990: Helping people to stop smoking: a study of the nurse's role. *Journal of Advanced Nursing* **15**, 357–63.

Macleod Clark, J., Wilson-Barnett, J., Latter, S. and Maben, J. 1992: *Health education and health promotion in nursing: a study of practice in acute areas*. Unpublished report of a two-year research project funded by the Department of Health. King's College, University of London, London.

McMahon, R. 1990: Power and collegial relations among nurses on wards adopting primary nursing and hierarchical ward management structures. *Journal of Advanced Nursing* **15**, 232–9.

Maglacas, A.M. 1988: Health For All: nursing's role. *Nursing Outlook* **36**, 66–71.

Manthey, M. 1992: *The practice of primary nursing.* London: King's Fund.

Parsons, T. 1951: *The social system.* London: Routledge and Kegan Paul.

Pearson, A. (ed.) 1988: *Primary nursing: nursing in the Burford and Oxford Nursing Development Units.* London: Croom Helm.

Rawson, D. and Grigg, C. 1988: *Purpose and practice in health education: the training and development needs of health education officers.* The Summary Report of the South Bank Health Education Research Project. London: South Bank University.

Rodwell, C.M. 1996: An analysis of the concept of empowerment. *Journal of Advanced Nursing* 2, 305–13.

Royal College of Nursing 1989: *Into the nineties: promoting professional excellence.* London: Royal College of Nursing.

Salvage, J. 1990: The theory and practice of the 'new Nursing'. *Nursing Times* 86, 42–5.

Salvage, J. 1992: The new nursing: empowering patients or empowering nurses? In Robinson, J. (ed.), *Policy issues in nursing.* Milton Keynes: Open University Press, 9–23.

Tones, K. 1991: Health promotion, empowerment and the psychology of control. *Journal of the Institute of Health Education* 29, 17–25.

Tones, K. 1993: The theory of health promotion: implications for nursing. In Wilson-Barnett, J. and Macleod Clark, J. (eds), *Research in health promotion and nursing.* Basingstoke: Macmillan, 3–12.

Tones, K. and Tilford, S. 1994: *Health education: effectiveness, efficiency and equity.* London: Chapman and Hall.

United Kingdom Central Council for Nurses, Midwives and Health Visitors 1986: *Project 2000.* London: United Kingdom Central Council for Nurses, Midwives and Health Visitors.

Waterworth, S. and Luker, K. 1990: Reluctant collaborators: do patients want to be involved in decisions concerning care? *Journal of Advanced Nursing* 15, 971–6.

Watts, R.J. 1990: Democratization of health care: challenge for nursing. *Advances in Nursing Science* 12, 37–46.

Weinstein, R. 1991: Hospital case management: the path to empowering nurses. *Pediatric Nursing* 17, 289–93

Williams, D. 1987: *Nursing and health promotion: contradictions between the goals of the profession and its model of health promotion.* Unpublished PhD Thesis, University of Delaware, Delaware.

Williams, D. 1989: Political theory and individualistic health promotion. *Advances in Nursing Science* 12, 14–25.

Williams, W. 1995: Education for empowerment: implications for professional development and training in health promotion. *Health Education Journal* 54, 37–47.

World Health Organization 1989: *Nursing Leadership for Health For All.* Geneva: World Health Organization Division of Health Manpower Development.

Wright, S. 1985: *Building and using a model of nursing.* London: Edward Arnold.

2

Implementing theory into primary health care practice: an empowering approach

Jackie Sturt

Introduction

As a consequence of both national and international political initiatives, the last decade has seen health promotion being placed high on the National Health Service agenda. These initiatives began internationally with the declaration of Alma Ata (World Health Organization, 1978) and nationally with the publication of *The Health of the Nation* (Department of Health, 1992). In many respects these two documents reflected contradictory approaches to the promotion of health. The former emphasized improvements in world health through the eradication of inequalities between and within countries, while the latter concentrated its efforts on epidemiological and lifestyle explanations for health differentials.

The health promotion literature aligns itself more closely with the World Health Organization's approach to improving world health, and has consequently focused substantially on the concept of empowerment as a mechanism for enabling individuals to address their own and others' health needs. Health professionals have therefore been presented with a dilemma associated with government policy and health funding organized around epidemiological targets and the recognition of the need to work enablingly with patients to address their own health concerns.

This chapter draws upon research undertaken by the author, and describes a study which attempted to address this need for primary health care practitioners to work in an enabling way with patients to address their health promotion needs. Action research was identified as an appropriate methodological approach for the qualitative exploration of health promotion and empowerment theory and the process of incorporating these into primary health care (PHC) practice. The chapter begins with an examination of the concept of empowerment as it relates to the practice of primary health care.

Bandura's (1977) self-efficacy theory was identified in the literature (Strecher *et al.*, 1986; Steele *et al.*, 1987; Gecas, 1989; Kendall, 1991a,b) as having the potential to inform the work of health professionals in an enabling way. Self-efficacy theory is defined and described with an emphasis on its relevance to empowering health promotion practice. Whilst self-efficacy theory has retained its potential for facilitating enabling work with patients, the study was hindered by the choice of smoking cessation as the health promotion priority for the primary health care team (PHCT). This chapter presents data from the study which indicates the potential of self-efficacy theory for informing an empowering approach to health promotion practice, whilst at the same time stressing a number of areas in which particular caution is required when practitioners implement the theory into their own practice.

Empowerment and primary health care

The publication of *The Health of the Nation* (Department of Health, 1992) placed health promotion firmly on the political agenda and gave primary health care a substantial role in addressing and achieving the health targets set by the government's policy. This policy identified five key areas where reductions in morbidity and mortality were to be made. The key areas were prescriptive, and recommendations for achieving change focused upon the formation of healthy alliances between health services providers, voluntary and leisure services, industry and commerce. Above all, responsibility was given to individuals to assess the impact of their lifestyle and health-related behaviour upon their own and their families' health and to make the necessary changes, with the appropriate help of health professionals. However, the political agenda established by *The Health of the Nation* was inconsistent with the ideology put forward by the health promotion literature (e.g. Tones, 1991; Labonte, 1994), which suggested the need for empowering approaches to health promotion, focusing on specific health needs indicated by population groups and individuals.

Tones (1991) suggested an approach to health promotion practice which could be focused upon individuals and on groups as members of a community, and proposed that each held equal value in the promotion of enabling health care practice.

> My proposals for the contribution of health education to the more broad concept of health promotion give pride of place to the complementary processes of critical consciousness raising and life-skills teaching as a major stratagem for the achievement of empowerment.
>
> (Tones, 1991, p. 25)

Labonte's 'Empowerment Holosphere' also advocated work within a number of spheres as a mechanism for reducing the disparities which existed between social groups. Labonte's personal care sphere relates to that area of activity at which most 'front-line' (Labonte, 1994, p. 259) health professionals work, and mirrors the area of health promotion activity in which Tones' (1991) life-skills training would take place. The health professional's individualistic focus, which this personal approach endorses, has been subjected to some criticism (e.g. Gott and O'Brien, 1990; Kendall, 1992), although it has been suggested by Dines (1994) that it is entirely intentional and appropriate that nurses work in this way as broader, more structural and community-oriented perspectives would prove to be beyond the scope of most nurses. Whilst this debate continues, the respective works of Tones (1991) and Labonte (1994) do establish a convincing rationale for working on a one-to-one basis with individuals, to address their health needs in an enabling way.

Action research, heavily influenced by the critical theorists Habermas (1972, 1974, 1979) and Freire (1972), informed the methodological approach to the implementation of a potentially empowering health promotion theory (self-efficacy theory; Bandura, 1977) into the individualized practitioner–patient health promotion encounters of a primary health care team.

Self-efficacy theory defined

Self-efficacy theory is concerned with an individual's perception of personal efficacy. Perceptions of efficacy determine whether or not individuals will first attempt an action or behaviour, and second the extent to which they will persevere in overcoming obstacles and finally be successful in the challenge.

Self-efficacy is measured in three parameters – level, strength, and generality. 'Level' refers to the individual's anticipated performance achievement, for example, 'I will be able to avoid smoking at home, but unable to avoid having a cigarette when in the pub'. 'Strength' is the individual's measure of confidence that he or she will attain the afore-mentioned level, for example, 'I am 80 per cent sure I can avoid smoking at home'. 'Generality' is the extent to which a person judges him- or herself to be efficacious in life generally, for example, 'I also believe that I could increase my level of exercise successfully, but I cannot successfully change my diet'.

Bandura (1977) identified outcome expectation as a second determinant of successful behaviour change, i.e. an individual's belief that a particular action will generate a particular and desirable outcome. Efficacy and outcome expectations are linked thus; individuals will act if they believe that their actions will lead to a personally desirable outcome (outcome

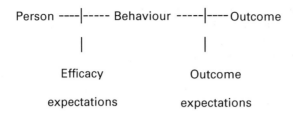

Person ----|----- Behaviour -----|---- Outcome

Efficacy   Outcome

expectations   expectations

Figure 2.1 The relationship between efficacy and outcome expectations; adapted from Bandura (1977), p. 193

expectation) and if they perceive themselves as having the necessary abilities to be reasonably sure of success (efficacy expectation). In Figure 2.1 the two concepts are placed on a person – behaviour – outcome chain.

For the individual, efficacy expectations play a role in determining whether he or she will engage in the new behaviour. Outcome expectations come into play when the individual appraises the potential new behaviour and decides whether that new behaviour will lead to a desirable outcome.

Bandura (1982) suggested that our self-efficacy judgements determine the choice of activities and behaviours in which we engage. This could prove to be useful as an explanatory theory accounting for the relative successes and failures of health promotion programmes on an individual basis. That is, perhaps failure is not always the fault of the programme in terms of style and content, but perhaps negative outcomes sometimes occur because some individuals respond well and others poorly, depending upon their individual perceptions of efficacy in that particular area.

Sources of efficacy information

According to Bandura (1977), the sources of information which formulate perceptions of personal efficacy are:

- performance accomplishments;
- vicarious experience;
- verbal persuasion;
- emotional arousal.

Bandura suggests that it is by intervention in these processes that efficacy enhancement may occur. Performance accomplishments are of most value and interest in that they are experiences of personal mastery of an action or behaviour. Succeeding in a challenge is said to increase an individual's perception of personal mastery, whereas failure will lower it. Repeated failures early on in experience can substantially lower mastery expectations, and thus self-efficacy expectations. However, once initial successes have been secured, an occasional failure which is subsequently overcome, can have a strengthening effect.

Vicarious experience is the process of observing others succeed or fail in their actions and behaviours. A great deal of personal efficacy information is derived in this manner. Seeing others, especially those of demographic similarity, performing given activities can increase the observer's efficacy perceptions of being able to perform similar actions him- or herself. Bandura suggested, however, that as vicarious experience relies so heavily on 'inferences from social comparison' (Bandura, 1977, p. 197), it remains less dependable as a source of efficacy expectation than performance accomplishments. Because of this, the behavioural outcomes are likely to be brittle and vulnerable to change.

Verbal persuasion is an over-used and over-rated tool in terms of successful efficacy enhancement. Efficacy expectations which have been acquired through verbal leadership alone are very much weaker than those which arise from personal mastery or vicarious experience. Bandura suggested that verbal persuasions lack the foundations of actual experience in that 'they do not provide an authentic experiential base' (Bandura, 1977, p. 198). It would also seem likely that the use of verbal persuasion alone as a source of efficacy information may account for a low success rate in performance accomplishment. If one repeatedly tries and fails, based upon social suggestion, this will lead to a downward spiralling of personal efficacy expectation and result in repeated failure as a direct consequence. Eventually the individual will no longer attempt the action, fully convinced of his or her inability to succeed.

Bandura did suggest a role for verbal persuasion when used in conjunction with modelling and participant modelling experiences:

> People who are socially persuaded that they possess the capabilities to master difficult situations and are provided with provisional aids for effective action are likely to mobilize greater effort than those who receive only the performance aids . . . It is therefore the interactive as well as the independent effects of social persuasion on self-efficacy that merit experimental consideration.
>
> (Bandura, 1977, p. 198)

Emotional arousal most commonly occurs when a person is faced with stressful or demanding situations, and it manifests itself in physiological symptoms, including sweating palms, short shallow breaths and palpitations. People rely on such physical cues as a signal of their level of emotional arousal, and this in turn becomes an indication of their competence, therefore providing efficacy information. A high level of arousal usually has a debilitating effect on performance. Consequently individuals are more likely to experience success when they are calm and relaxed.

In his seminal paper on self-efficacy Bandura (1977) suggested however, that these four sources of efficacy information do not occur in isolation, and depend on how the information received is cognitively appraised by the individual. A number of other factors will influence whether, for example, a successful mastery experience is cognitively processed as occurring as a result of the individual's own efforts, or whether they believe they were successful for reasons peculiar to the situation, such as involvement with a therapist or in a laboratory. Similarly, the effects of verbal persuasion can be determined by the credibility of the second person involved in the interaction. Bandura thus identified and drew together a number of mechanisms through which perceptions of efficacy might become subject to enhancement.

Self-efficacy theory as an empowering framework for health-promoting practice

The discipline of health promotion asserts that inequalities in health can only be addressed by approaches to health promotion work which are enabling and empowering for individuals (e.g. Tones, 1991; Labonte, 1994; Benzeval *et al.*, 1995). Gecas suggested that low perceptions of personal efficacy and powerlessness are synonymous: research indicates that high self-efficacy has beneficial and therapeutic consequences for individuals and low self-efficacy (powerlessness) has negative and maladaptive consequences (Gecas, 1989, p. 298).

This represents a potentially strong framework for helping individuals along the continuum from powerlessness to powerfulness via the process of efficacy enhancement. The nature of self-efficacy theory ensures a focus on the specific identification of problematic areas for the individual which, using Gecas's (1989) argument, would involve a focus on areas where they experience a degree of powerlessness. The tools used in the measurement of efficacy perceptions relate directly and unavoidably to the individual's experience. They remain the information source for the assessment of efficacy perceptions, and enhancement can only be successful if it is based specifically upon this assessment. A self-efficacy framework for practice is something which cannot be performed on an individual; it necessitates his or her full involvement and control. The individual controls the health agenda, the measurement and, as a consequence of the fact that he or she is the one performing it, the efficacy enhancement. In this way, a self-efficacy framework provides an opportunity to enhance perceptions of efficacy which will reduce both the perception and the experience of powerlessness.

Self-efficacy theory has been suggested as being theoretically linked, as a determinant, to active patienthood. Steele *et al.* (1987) reviewed the literature in relation to the active patient concept and summarized their findings by suggesting that further research needed to be undertaken to elaborate upon the links between active patient participation and self-regulatory theories of health behaviour such as self-efficacy theory. They went on to recommend clinically that efficacy expectations be accounted for in treatment programming: 'Clinicians would be well advised to assess their patients' illness representations and self-efficacy perceptions and tailor treatment to these perceptions' (Steele *et al.*, 1987, p. 19).

Strecher *et al.* (1986) distinguished self-efficacy theory from other models and theories of health behaviour change when they identified a similar potential in the theory. They used Bartlett (1983) to illustrate their hypothesis pertaining to its potential in relation to patient participation: 'Self-efficacy provides the theoretical buttress for the notion of the activated patient.' (Bartlett, 1983, p. 547, cited in Strecher, 1986, p. 89.)

From a health-visiting perspective, Kendall (1991b) was encouraged by self-efficacy theory on the basis that it appeared to hold the potential for encouraging client participation at a time when such participation in health visiting practice was being professionally advocated. From the perspective of the practitioner, Kendall demonstrated the capacity of the theory to begin and end with the patient:

> Bandura's theory offers a framework in which client participation can preside because it takes as its starting point the perceived self-efficacy of the client. If the health visitor is able to assess the extent to which a patient feels able to cope with a situation and then take action, then care planning will, of necessity, start from the client's point of view rather than that of the health visitor, whose own perception of the situation might be very different.
>
> (Kendall, 1991b, p. 9)

Health promotion practice theoretically linked to self-efficacy theory might enable practitioners to continue to work in a patient-focused and individual way, whilst maintaining an emphasis on both the lifestyle and the socio-cultural context of the patient's life. Within a particular health area, it would emphasize the patient's agenda rather than that of the professional, and enable the patient to begin to take control of the consultation and the processes and objectives which emerge from it. In this way the individual can engage in the empowering process, which might begin with control over the pace at which they work, and proceed to the establishment of greater control over their own life.

These perspectives, from the literature, on the importance of empowerment in the promotion of health provided this study with the theoretical validity for participating with a primary health care team in the implementation of self-efficacy theory into their health promotion practice.

Introduction to the study

Research access was negotiated with an urban primary health care team in southern England to explore the process of implementing health promotion theory (self-efficacy theory) into the health promotion work engaged in by team members. The study used an action research approach informed by critical theory (Carr and Kemmis, 1986; Hart and Bond, 1995). Six members of the PHCT (one general practitioner, three practice nurses and two health visitors) sustained their commitment and interest in the study throughout a 12-month period. The six remaining members of the team participated less frequently. The PHCT identified smoking cessation as the health promotion priority on which they wished to concentrate their initial efforts, as part of the research process.

The research questions were as follows. *Can self-efficacy theory inform health promotion practice in a primary health care team? Can emancipatory action research facilitate critical thinking and the conscientization of a primary health care team?* (The latter research question is discussed in Sturt, 1997). The research aims centred around understanding the processes of changing practice and qualitative outcomes. Thus, for example, demonstrating reductions in the smoking incidence in the practice population was not relevant to the research question. The self-efficacy framework for smoking cessation which arose from this study is the focus of the discussion surrounding the relevance of the theory as a potential health promotion tool for practice. The relevance of the health promotion message and the role of outcome expectations will be scrutinized to provide further discussion on the effectiveness of health promotion using this approach.

The use of self-efficacy theory in primary health care: the potential for health promotion practice

The validity of self-efficacy theory as an effective theoretical framework within which to base health promotion practice has been evaluated within the literature (e.g. O'Leary, 1985; Strecher *et al.*, 1986; Kasen *et al.*, 1992). By using an instrument to measure perceptions of efficacy (e.g. Nicki *et al.*, 1984; Hickey *et al.*, 1992; Kasen *et al.*, 1992), it is possible to identify those individuals who are most likely to initiate and sustain new health-related behaviours. This study sought to take this established theoretical approach and to facilitate its application in the practice setting of a professional group for whom health promotion theory has remained elusive. In doing so, it was important to identify the process of implementation and to establish those aspects of the framework which were significant for the primary health care team in their learning, development of practice and utilization of the framework.

It is acknowledged that the factors which existed for this primary health care team are highly specific and contextually related. There were, however, a great many similarities, relating to the health promotion practice of this team, with the work of the practitioners described in the studies by Gott and O'Brien (1990), Macleod Clark *et al.* (1992) and Latter (1994). This would suggest that the constraints to enabling practice are more broadly experienced within health promotion nursing.

Self-efficacy as facilitating patient control

One of the strengths of self-efficacy theory, as an appropriate health promotion framework, was the degree to which it was suggested as facilitating patient control in a health context (Bartlett, 1983; Steele *et al.*, 1987; Gecas, 1989; Kendall, 1991b). Patient control is linked to the active patient concept and, in this context, refers to the extent to which patients control both the health agenda and the manner in which it is addressed. This, together with claims that health promotion practice needed to be enabling (e.g.Tones, 1991; Department of Health, 1992; Labonte, 1994), led to a research initiative which linked enabling health promotion practice and self-efficacy theory. Self-efficacy theory held the potential for practitioner use, to enable them to orientate their practice towards this goal.

Whilst the data provided a great deal of evidence to illustrate the more disempowering side of health professional–patient encounters, analysis of the data demonstrated occasions when both individual team members and the team as a whole were able to surrender control to the patient during consultations, illustrating the degree to which self-efficacy theory held the potential for a high level of patient participation.

The practitioners' use of the framework, nevertheless, made it essential that the consultation rested heavily upon the patient and his or her perceptions and goals, however specifically oriented to smoking or weight loss. The following data extract illustrates the case of a particularly controlling practice nurse (PN1), as demonstrated by her consistent use of both instructive and prescriptive advice to patients, as effectively and creatively using the framework to help patients to address their smoking behaviour:

JS: *How do you feel about your successes?*

PN1: *Well I'm delighted when they cut down, but the last [patient] was so difficult and we had to abandon the questionnaire completely because she was totally different to anyone I had met giving up cigarettes. Because she smoked in the most odd way.*

PN1 described how the patient had smoked 20 cigarettes a day, but was not allowed to smoke at work, and smoked almost all of those cigarettes from five o'clock onwards in the evening. On completing the questionnaire, the patient maintained that she could resist most of the situations because she did so during the day at work. The nurse continued;

PN1: *I had a terrible job to get her to smoke one cigarette at lunchtime, and timing her in the end. I said 'You must time your cigarettes,' I said 'You can't smoke more than one cigarette an hour.' It was half an hour to start off with and then an hour . . . she gave up [smoking] in the end.*

I asked PN1 whether they had identified different situations for the patient in degrees of difficulty:

PN1: *Oh yes she did, we had a list for her, a list completely separate, there was nothing on the formal questionnaire that dealt with her, she was very odd ... and in the end I was very strict and said look you cannot smoke more than one cigarette in an hour and I said 'Put your alarm clock on if necessary, otherwise,' I said, 'you're not going to manage.' And she did, she cut down from 10 cigarettes then nine then eight then two.*

Whilst PN1 maintained a controlling manner in her dialogue with the patient, there is evidence that the consultation, guided by the self-efficacy framework, focused upon the patient's perspective of the problem. The use of time limits provided a strategy for sequential goal achievement with a patient who otherwise failed to fit into the normal situational pattern. The use of self-efficacy theory to guide the consultation overrode PN1's prescriptive and controlling manner.

This close adherence to the patient's experience in the design of a smoking cessation programme can be identified in GP1's work with a male patient in his late twenties:

GP1: *We looked at the various areas, and we talked about the life he has got, a girlfriend who is supportive, she would like him to give up, he would like to give up. He recognises that one of his problems is that he is a keen cricketer and all his cricket mates [smoke], so if he is going to tackle it he is going to have to come to terms with going out for drinks with his mates, he thinks that is going to be the hardest. In fact, if you look at his scores, in pubs and things, he doesn't do quite so well.*

He has told his girlfriend and all his friends that he is going to stop ... after he has settled into his new job ... So we thought we would try working through the various areas ... so we started with his car, he went away for a week, put cigarettes in his boot, cleaned his car, chewing gum ... and he went away and it worked, he played a lot of music and ate a lot of chewing gum ... so he was very pleased, genuinely very pleased.

GP1 continued to describe to his colleagues the details of his patient's life and smoking behaviour. There is a strong feeling of negotiated activity in GP1's descriptions in his use of 'we' throughout. These excerpts provide an illustration of the extent to which links were made between the patients' perceptions of their smoking behaviour and its context, and the theoretical approach to cessation provided by self-efficacy.

The data analysis demonstrates that when the health promotion priorities of both patient and practitioner coincide, the use of self-efficacy theory to guide the health promotion consultation is able to provide an appropriately patient-focused consultation which goes further than a mere assessment of the behaviour. The self-efficacy framework for practice insists upon a broad understanding of the pertinent contextual reality for the patient related to a given behaviour. As a result, the *self-efficacy-informed consultation* appeared to play a more significant role in health promotion practice than did the personal practice style of the health professional.

Where there was agreement between patient and health professional on the patient's health needs, the self-efficacy framework facilitated a substantial degree of patient participation and control. Where there was not such agreement, the practitioners were unable to shift their emphasis away from their smoking priority focus to engage with the patients in their own agenda. In this respect, the experience of using the self-efficacy framework distanced it from the ideas which had originally linked it to an empowering approach to health promotion work. Kendall (1991a) found that health visitors did not use enabling strategies in their consultations with mothers, and suggested that the use of a theoretical framework to guide practice might promote the use of client participation. This research shows that this is only the case where the identified needs of the patient are addressed. This attempt to use an enabling health promotion approach to address perceived health needs which did not actually belong to the patient was unable to foster the patients' interest in the health promotion agenda being pursued.

The relevance of having an appropriate health promotion message

An important point to emerge from the experience of self-efficacy implementation surrounds the need to identify the patient's real health priorities. The practitioners reported and demonstrated that, for the majority of smoking patients with whom they engaged, smoking cessation was of little interest. The smoking priority had emerged as a general practitioner-led idea with the other discipline groups, with the exception of the practice nurses, having identified other concerns when asked to present an experientially based analysis of health needs as pertinent to their practice caseload. The GPs' smoking emphasis was identified and substantiated by its potential for health gain, were the project to be successful in improving the outcomes of health promotion work in the practice. Despite the statistical evidence presented to the team, which showed smoking figures consistent with the national average and, for example, an incidence of raised body mass index (BMI) in certain age groups exceeding the national average, very little discussion arose from it, and the subsequent health prioritization discussion within the disciplinary groups made no reference to it. Where patient interest occurred, the measurement of perceptions of efficacy and subsequent enhancement provided encouragement for the professional involved and demonstrated the validity of the framework for health promotion practice in primary health care. The lack of patient interest which led to the disappointment and frustration subsequently experienced by team members demonstrates the inappropriateness of the smoking cessation priority. What this suggests for the process of implementing health promotion theory, in this particular instance self-efficacy theory, is that the appropriateness of the priority for those on the receiving end of service provision will determine the degree of their engagement in the health behaviour change.

From the perspective of implementing self-efficacy theory as a framework for practice, it would therefore appear essential to approach health promotion priorities from the perspective of the patient, and not from the perspective of a general practice agenda based upon political and fiscal imperatives. This would entail one of two things – either a community-led prioritization process which aimed to seek the views of the practice population (e.g. Adams, 1995; Thomas, 1996), or an individually based approach which would seek to discuss a broad range of health needs with every patient with whom a health professional came into opportunistic contact. Having established the highest health priority, this would entail organizing a service based upon providing help for patients to achieve their objectives in relation to their personal goals, using the self-efficacy framework to guide the process.

Once the primary concerns for a given patient were established, a self-efficacy framework for practice could help that patient to address his or her own individual health requirements. Whilst the latter method might be more appealing to nurses, based upon the evidence relating to their unique interest in the individual patient (e.g. Gott and O'Brien, 1990; Latter, 1994), it would necessitate a comprehensive knowledge of the self-efficacy literature, especially in relation to measurement scales for the assessment of efficacy perceptions. Nurses are recognized for their interest in working with, and effectiveness of access to, the individual patient. In the light of the work of Tones (1991) and Labonte (1994) on the appropriateness of both a personal and a community orientation towards enabling and empowering health promotion practice, this might suggest that resources are best directed at the potential of nursing work to continue in an individually focused manner, rather than have nursing practice reoriented towards a community action perspective. If health promotion nursing practice is to continue in its present form, resources must also go into the process of developing awareness amongst nurses regarding the socio-economic consequences of the lives of the patients whom they see.

The low levels of patient interest in the smoking cessation priority made a significant contribution to the waning enthusiasm of the practitioners to engage further in this study. As a result, this health promotion research initiative succeeded in developing a self-efficacy practice framework which was exposed to limited evaluation. The evidence which does relate to the effectiveness of the framework to inform practice is nevertheless encouraging, as one of PN1's experiences illustrates:

PN1: *I re-tested my lady this week and it is very interesting. She says she still cannot cope in the morning without that one cigarette.*

HV1: *That's the first thing she does is it?*

PN1: *Not now, she drags it out for over an hour and a bit, she doesn't smoke for over an hour first thing.*

JS: *Still she has gone from a 3 to an 8* [reference to self-efficacy score].

PN1:   *Whereas it was the first thing she did when she got up, she is trying to rush herself so that she hasn't got time to smoke, but she says she cannot cope without that one cigarette.*

HV1:   *That's very good, look at all those 10s.*

PN1:   *She has come down from 20 a day, she has done very well.*

This scenario indicates, in both psychological and behavioural ways, the impact made on the patient's smoking activity by the self-efficacy approach to cessation. The self-efficacy score increased from 3 to 8, suggesting that her confidence in resisting that morning cigarette was high but not complete. In addition, the scores are substantiated by PN1's knowledge of the patient's actual behaviour, having reduced from 20 cigarettes a day to just one.

The evidence reinforces the view that health promotion initiatives necessitate the sustained commitment of health professionals, and it recognizes the importance of identifying health promotion priorities which will sustain the interest of the patient population being served. It cannot be assumed, however, that this will be an easy process. The experience of Thomas (1996) suggested that, to her surprise, many members of the GP practice population to which she addressed her health needs assessment declined to participate. Nevertheless, the exercise has to assume importance if health promotion work in PHC is to be effective in improving the health of practice populations.

Format for the development of trust in the theory

The development of trust in self-efficacy theory, and the developing framework for health promotion practice, can be identified as an essential feature of the process of implementation. Three factors characterized and contributed significantly to increasing the trustworthiness of the framework for the team. These were a *cognitive understanding of the consultation format*, the *production of a strategy list* to aid the practitioners whilst engaged in the consultation, and finally *an outcome measure in the form of altered health behaviour*.

A cognitive understanding of the consultation format was facilitated by providing the team with multiple opportunities to rehearse the format for patient consultations using self-efficacy theory. The rehearsal and subsequent execution of self-efficacy consultations was significant in developing team mastery in the use of self-efficacy theory. It provided those involved in the rehearsal with mastery experiences, and for those team members who were listening and offering ideas it provided the vicarious experience. Bandura *et al.*'s (1980) description of cognitive modelling and the development of cognitive mastery offers one possible explanation regarding the significance of the consultation rehearsals for the development of both confidence and skill in using the framework. The process involved in the enhancement of efficacy perceptions by cognitive modelling is not dissimilar to that experienced by the practitioners as they questioned and described the consultation format. Bandura *et al.* (1980) demonstrated that cognitive mastery of threats enhanced the perceptions of personal efficacy and this, as with the present study, went on to predict the performance attainment of the participants when presented with the real threat. The cognitive imagery which occurred as a consequence of the consultation rehearsals can be identified as significant, as trust and confidence in the framework evolved.

The *production of the strategy list* was significant at a number of levels. Initially its value lay in its use as an *aide-mémoire* during the consultation. It represented an addition to the professional health promotion tool kit, about which the practitioner could feel secure when in need of an idea. In addition, the process of its construction reveals something of the nature of the participants. During its early construction, attempts to utilize the information were being geared very much towards a universal form to hand out to patients in a non-specific manner. When it became clear that its use should be tailored more individually to patients, it became a potent source of information which afforded the health professional extra power over the process of the consultation because they retained knowledge which the patient then had to request from them. By the point in the implementation when the self-efficacy framework was established and rehearsed, and confidence in its use was strong, the strategy list became an example of the team's ability to be patient centred. Whilst there were few general similarities between a Tones' (1991) or a Labonte's (1994) description of enabling practice and that described by the practitioners via their critical incidents, they none the less saw the strategy list as a resource to enable them to address the sharing of control between themselves and the patients, demonstrating a willingness to support their patients. Whilst there is little evidence within the data that a characteristic of the consultation was its empowering nature, there is evidence – as discussed above – that the use of the self-efficacy framework for practice did contribute to a patient focus during consultations, despite the controlling tendencies of some practitioners. The strategy list could have been a significant feature of this focusing, and have demonstrated to the practitioner the efficacy of sharing control, thus becoming identified as an enabling device.

The research outcomes were about understanding the process of changing practice, and demonstrable outcomes, e.g. in smoking cessation, were not relevant to the research questions. However, the collection of data in the form of critical incidents, discussed both individually and within a group format, identified some patients who had been helped to stop smoking via the practitioners' use of self-efficacy theory to guide the process. The *production of an outcome measure in the form of altered behaviour* was of substantial efficacy-enhancing value for the practitioners concerned. The experience of going through a smoking cessation exercise with a patient and demonstrating a change in their smoking behaviour, both by the measurement of efficacy expectations and in actual behavioural terms in their decreasing levels of reported smoking, was confidence building for the practitioners. Not only did it influence the degree of trust with which they viewed the theoretical framework, but also they were able to trust their own abilities in facilitating the process. The observation of altered smoking behaviour that team members experienced can be seen as significant in the context of this study, as it represents one of the few occasions when a meeting point occurred between efficacy and outcome expectations (Bandura, 1977).

The role of outcome expectations

One of the areas in which self-efficacy theory (Bandura,1977) has been subjected to theoretical criticism has been in the field of understanding and accounting for outcome expectations (Gecas, 1989). Indeed, the role of outcome expectations has, in this study, played a more significant role in explaining some of the research processes than it did in the development of the self-efficacy framework. In the framework development, the only outcome expectations which the team had identified and considered were those associated with the health benefits derived from smoking cessation. This outcome expectation had been addressed by acknowledging the need to target efforts in the direction of motivated patients. The motivated status of the patient would indicate that they expected that stopping smoking would result in improvements in their health status. Ongoing analysis of the research process and the formal data analysis revealed a number of factors for which consideration of the role of outcome expectations can provide an explanation.

The level of patient disinterest in the smoking cessation orientation of the study validates the need to consider, as the primary health care team (PHCT) did, the relevance of outcome expectations. This disinterest may relate to patients' disbelief that stopping smoking would lead to improvements in health. Alternatively, it may relate to the patients' expectation that if they were to engage in the process, they would continue to smoke, i.e. the programme would not work for them. In reviewing smoking cessation intervention in GP practice, the OXCHECK (Imperial Cancer Research Fund, 1995) study questioned the value of the brief intervention smoking cessation practice among GPs, suggesting that the results of Russell *et al.* (1979), which indicated that the brief advice method was efficacious, related to a very different smoking population: 'As the prevalence of smoking has fallen, the proportion of smokers who can relinquish the habit with information and support alone has most certainly fallen' (Imperial Cancer Research Fund, 1995, p. 1102). If this is the case, the established smokers who remain are most likely to be those for whom smoking cessation attempts have previously failed. An experience of failure would have left them with lowered confidence both in their own ability to stop smoking (efficacy expectations) and in the efficacy of any method designed to help them (outcome expectations). This was a patient outcome expectation which the PHCT and I failed to consider as contributing to the low levels of interest in the study.

The role of outcome expectations can also provide an explanation for some of the issues which arose for the PHCT. For the health professional involved in the study, outcome expectations associated with improvements in their health promotion practice were positive during the early stages. Moreover, there were expectations of high levels of patient interest in the study. However, the experience of *actual* patient disinterest was clearly linked to dwindling practitioner interest as the study progressed, and thus it is pertinent to discuss the nature of the health professionals' changing expectations of outcome. As it became clear that few patients were attracted to the study, the team began to explore alternative health promotion priorities, returning to the ideas indicated by practitioner groups during an earlier practice awayday. Whilst there was sufficient enthusiasm to meet and discuss the way forward, resultant activity was minimal. The participants' view of the process suggests that the team considered self-efficacy theory to be responsible for the perceived failure of the study;

> PN2: *It gives the professional an awful sense of failure doesn't it? Because you think you're not getting the message across.*

> GP1: *The satisfaction or 'delight' that the self-efficacy theory brings to the health professional. I think [absence of delight] is its main failing . . . Unfortunately, in practice at some point during the supportive phase the patients just fail to attend. This may be because they have lost faith in the procedure or it may be that they have reverted to their previous health state.*

This situation contributed to the alteration of outcome expectations regarding self-efficacy theory. The practitioners ceased to believe in its potential for guiding their health promotion practice, since it had predominantly become associated with failure. Whilst on an individual level practitioners had experienced success in using the framework, the larger and more overwhelming picture was one of disappointment and failure. This resulted in a reluctance to participate enthusiastically within the context of another set of priority health needs. It is therefore possible that efficacy and outcome expectations might be linked in the following way. For these practitioners, being denied mastery experiences in the smoking cessation programme lowered their personal efficacy expectations of being able to achieve mastery in a diet or sexual health programme. Thus, contrary to Bandura's (1977) thesis, a degree of generality in the lowering of efficacy perceptions may have occurred. This may have reinforced their altered outcome expectations of the self-efficacy framework, establishing it as being unable to satisfy the team's outcome expectations, and so rendering it inappropriate for their practice.

On an individual level, where practitioner mastery experiences were evident, the contribution made by outcome expectations to the efficacy of the framework can be established. The study began with practitioners holding the outcome expectation that, by using self-efficacy theory, they would be more successful in helping patients to stop smoking. Where this occurred, and patients worked successfully through the programme, there was a demonstrable effect on the practitioner's confidence in the framework. On these occasions, positive mastery experiences provided a meeting place for both efficacy and outcome expectations which augmented the practitioners' confidence in the theory as an appropriate practice tool.

This study has demonstrated the importance of outcome expectations in the use of self-efficacy theory. Furthermore, it suggests, that a wide net needs to be cast by both practitioners and researchers when considering ideas and activities which have attributable outcomes and for which an expectation is established. This study did not recognize the need to consider outcome expectations comprehensively. This led to a dysfunction in the way in which self-efficacy theory could contribute to health promotion practice. Whilst the developed framework clearly demonstrates its effectiveness where the health needs analysis of practitioner and patient coincide, the outcome expectations of all participants and researchers need to be scrutinized in order that these can be built into, and addressed as part of, the qualitative research process.

Conclusions

This study demonstrated that self-efficacy theory has the potential for positively informing the health promotion practice of practitioners working in primary health care. The development and implementation of the theory was relatively simple for the practitioners involved, and offered a sound basis for a more patient-centred approach to health promotion. Thus self-efficacy theory represents an appropriate practice framework for PHCTs, with minimal resource implications of introducing the framework into practice. Competent use of the self-efficacy framework was facilitated by the utilization of cognitive modelling techniques (Bandura *et al.*, 1980). These took the form of extensive discussion surrounding the format of hypothetical patient consultations. Cognitive mastery of the use of the framework was supported by the mastery experiences afforded by actual patient encounters.

Two issues need to be seriously considered in order to maximize the potential of the framework. First, it is crucial to identify the real health priorities of the population to be served. The data demonstrated the potential for self-efficacy theory to address health issues only when the needs of the patients concurred with the services offered by the practitioners. Second, the outcome expectations of all of the participants need to be broadly considered and built into the implementation process. In this study, failure to do this resulted in the implementation process being inadvertently sabotaged by the respective expectations of outcome. If these points are built into the implementation of self-efficacy theory into health promotion practice, a sound framework exists for the exploration and enhancement of efficacy expectations.

References

Adams, S. 1995: The development of a team approach to health needs analysis in primary health care. Unpublished report submitted for a Smith & Nephew Nursing Fellowship. London: Smith & Nephew.

Bandura, A. 1977: Self-efficacy theory: toward a unifying theory of behaviour change. *Psychological Review* **84**, 191–215.

Bandura, A. 1982: Self-efficacy mechanisms in human agency. *American Psychologist* **37**, 122–47.

Bandura, A., Adams, N., Hardy, A. and Howells, G.N. 1980: Tests of the generality of self-efficacy theory. *Cognitive Therapy and Research* **4**, 39–66.

Bartlett, E. 1983: Educational self-help approaches in childhood asthma. *Journal of Allergy and Clinical Immunology* **72**, 545–53.

Benzeval, M., Judge, K. and Whitehead, M. 1995: Tackling inequalities in health: an agenda for action. London: The King's Fund.

Carr, W. and Kemmis, S. 1986: *Becoming critical: education, knowledge and action research.* London: The Falmer Press.

Department of Health 1992: *The Health of the Nation: a strategy for health in England.* London: HMSO.

Dines, A. 1994: What changes in health behaviour might nurses logically expect from their health promotion work? *Journal of Advanced Nursing* **20**, 219–26.

Freire, P. 1972: *Pedagogy of the oppressed.* Harmondsworth: Penguin.

Gecas, V. 1989: The social psychology of self-efficacy. *Annual Review of Sociology* **15**, 291–316.

Gott, M. and O'Brien, M. 1990: *The role of the nurse in health promotion: policies, perspectives and practice.* Milton Keynes: Department of Health and Social Welfare, The Open University.

Habermas, J. 1972: *Knowledge and human interests* (trans. J.J. Shapiro). London: Heinemann.

Habermas, J. 1974: *Theory and practice* (trans. J. Viertel). London: Heinemann.

Habermas, J. 1979: *Communication and the evolution of society.* Boston, MA: Beacon Press.

Hart, E. and Bond, M. 1995: *Action research for health and social care.* Oxford: Oxford University Press.

Hickey, M.L., Owens, S.V. and Froman, R.D. 1992: Instrument development: cardiac diet and exercise self-efficacy. *Nursing Research* **41**, 347–51.

Imperial Cancer Research Fund 1995: Effectiveness of health check conducted by nurses in primary care: final results of the OXCHECK study. *British Medical Journal* **310**, 1099–104.

Kasen, S.,Vaughan, R.D. and Walter, H.J. 1992: Self-efficacy for AIDS preventive behaviors among tenth-grade students. *Health Education Quarterly* **19**, 187–202.

Kendall, S.A. 1991a: *An analysis of the health visitor–client interaction: the influence of the health visiting process on client participation.* Unpublished PhD Thesis, King's College, University of London, London.

Kendall, S.A. 1991b: A home visit by the health visitor using Bandura's theory of self-efficacy. In White, A. (ed.), *Caring for children – towards partnership with families.* London: Edward Arnold, 4–14.

Kendall, J. 1992: Fighting back: promoting emancipatory nursing actions. *Advances in Nursing Science* **15**, 1–15.

Labonte, M.A. 1994: Health promotion and empowerment: reflections on professional practice. *Health Education Quarterly* **21**, 253–68.

Latter, S. 1994: *Health education and health promotion: perceptions and practice of nurses in acute care settings.* Unpublished PhD Thesis, King's College, University of London, London.

Macleod Clark, J., Wilson-Barnett, J., Latter, S. and Maben, J. 1992: *Health education and health promotion in nursing: a study of practice in acute areas.* Unpublished Department of Health-funded report. King's College, University of London, London.

Nicki, R.M., Remmington, R.E. and MacDonald, G.A. 1984: Self-efficacy, nicotine-fading/self-monitoring and cigarette-smoking behavior. *Behavior Research and Therapy* **22**, 477–85.

O'Leary, A. 1985: Self-efficacy and health. *Behaviour Research and Therapy* **23**, 437–51.

Russell, M.H., Wilson, C., Taylor, C. and Barker, C.D. 1979: Effect of general practitioners' advice against smoking. *British Medical Journal* **2**, 231–5.

Steele, D.J., Blackwell, B., Gutmann, M.C. and Jackson, T.C. 1987: The activated patient: dogma, dream or desideratum? Beyond advocacy: a review of the active patient concept. *Patient Education and Counselling* **10**, 3–23.

Strecher, V.J., McEnvoy De Villis, B., Becker, M.H. and Rosenstock, I. 1986: The role of self-efficacy in achieving health behaviour change. *Health Education Quarterly* **13**, 74–92.

Sturt, J.A. 1997: *The implementation of self-efficacy theory into health promotion practice in primary health care: an action research approach.* Unpublished PhD Thesis, Buckinghamshire Chilterns University College, Brunel University, Uxbridge.

Thomas, A. 1996: Assessing need. In Bryar, R. and Bytheway, B. (eds), *Changing primary health care: the Team Care Valley's Experience.* Oxford: Blackwell Science.

Tones, K. 1991: Health promotion, empowerment and the psychology of control. *Journal of the Institute Health Education* **29**, 17–26.

World Health Organization 1978: *Alma Ata Declaration.* Copenhagen: World Health Organization Regional Office for Europe.

3

Health education and the promotion of health: seeking wisely to empower

Keith Tones

Introduction

Although not without its critics (see, for instance, LeFanu, 1994), health promotion has enjoyed a good deal of popularity in recent time. It even figures prominently in the first 'official' national health policy document produced in England (Department of Health, 1992). None the less, health promotion is an essentially contested concept – it has a whole variety of meaning from which people can pick and choose at will! Accordingly, one of the main concerns of the present chapter is to provide a critical assessment of this multifaceted notion – primarily by focusing on the influential definition provided by World Health Organization (WHO).

This discussion of health promotion will centre on the dynamic interaction of health education and health policy and, in reviewing different 'models' of health education, will argue that ethically and practically the main goal of the educational endeavour should be empowerment. It will be argued that the empowerment strategy helps to resolve an important dilemma in health promotion – the need on the one hand to prevent disease and safeguard the public health, while on the other hand respecting individual freedom of choice, including the freedom to adopt an 'unhealthy' lifestyle.

For reasons of economy, the major focus of this chapter will be on health education rather than the equally relevant domain of policy development and implementation. We shall, in this context, assert that progress in the development of effective health education programmes will depend on the systematic application of theory to the proper design of community-wide initiatives. Underlying this assertion is the equally confident observation that health education does in fact have a substantial and sophisticated body of theory on which to draw! A brief overview will be provided of the major features of a theory-based systematic approach to efficient programme planning.

In all this we acknowledge that, as in politics, health promotion is replete with rhetoric! We shall therefore seek to demonstrate how the rhetoric of empowerment might be operationalized and applied in the primary care context.

Finally, we shall explore the much debated issue of the effectiveness and efficiency of health education. We shall ask what we mean by success. We shall point out that success will depend on the synergistic application of the right methods in the right place at the right time, and will indicate the kinds of indicators which health educators might use to demonstrate their effectiveness and efficiency. We shall conclude by stating with some equanimity that health education can indeed be effective and, moreover, that it should be provided for people as a right.

Health promotion: anatomy and ideology

The term 'ideology' is used here in its simplest form, and merely describes the complex of values inherent in belief systems and underpinning personal and professional practice. The conceptualization of health promotion in this chapter incorporates the ideological canons of the WHO which are central to its *Health for All by the Year 2000* (HFA 2000) initiative and embodied in many landmark developments, such as primary health care (PHC) and the Ottawa Charter (World Health Organization, 1986). The ethical and moral view of humanity enshrined in the WHO's perspective may be summarized as follows.

- Health should be viewed holistically. It is a positive state and an essential commodity which people need in order to achieve a socially and economically productive life.
- Health will not be achieved nor illness prevented and controlled unless existing health inequalities between and within nations and social groups have been eradicated.
- A healthy nation is not only one which has an equitable distribution of resources, but also one which has active empowered communities which are vigorously involved in creating the conditions necessary for a healthy people.
- Health is too important to be left to medical practitioners; there must be a 'reorientation of health services'. It is also important to recognize that a wide range of public and private services and institutions influence health for good or ill. Moreover, medical services frequently do not meet the needs of the public; they often treat people as passive recipients of care and are thus fundamentally depowering. The main *modus operandi* of health promotion is one of enabling not coercing. The focus should be on co-operation rather than on compliance.

- People's health is not just an individual responsibility. Our health is to a large extent governed by the physical, social, cultural and economic environments in which we live and work. To cajole people into taking responsibility for their health, while at the same time ignoring the social and environmental circumstances which conspire to make them ill, is a fundamentally defective strategy – and unethical. It is, in short, victim-blaming. For these reasons, the process of 'building healthy public policy' is at the very heart of health promotion (from Tones and Tilford, 1994, pp. 4–5).

The five canons of health promotion theology listed above can receive only cursory consideration in this chapter. However, two observations are appropriate at this juncture. First of all, the list of principles is an intriguing mix of verifiable fact and value judgement. On the one hand there is quite clearly an inequitable distribution of both resources and health – and an undoubted interaction between the two. Health is influenced by a wide variety of services other than the 'traditional' medical services. Government policy quite manifestly influences a nation's health status for good or ill. Moreover, we should note the WHO's change in emphasis from its original constitutional declaration that health and well-being represent an ultimate desirable state. It now asserts that the desirable endpoint is a socially and economically productive life – and it must surely be true that ill health acts as a barrier to the attainment of these twin goals at both an individual and a societal level.

On the other hand, the ideological components contained in the five principles are contestable. Why should health be viewed holistically or as a positive state? Why should people not be subjected to authoritarian regimes and cajoled and coerced into compliance with medical advice? Should individuals and communities really be empowered? Would it not be better for them to put themselves into the hands of their chosen deity or to succumb to the benevolent dicta of their rulers – or malevolent destiny?

Readers will doubtless recognize some areas of current political contention in the questions raised above. Interestingly, while these questions would be of the rhetorical variety for those committed to the WHO school of health promotion, they would represent points of real political concern for many of a right-wing conviction who might well find themselves entangled in a number of conflicting value judgements. The implementation of healthy public policy which obliges people to be healthy will give rise to complaints about the 'nanny state' limiting individual freedom and enterprise. By contrast, talk of empowerment has an unpleasant ring of left-wing revolutionary movements!

The second observation to be made about the WHO's major health promotion principles is that, since they were incorporated in the Ottawa Charter (World Health Organization, 1986), a majority of nations – including the UK government – have apparently committed themselves to these principles as signatories of the Charter!

Health promotion: the contribution of education

There is still, in some quarters, a degree of uncertainty about the difference between health education and health promotion. For some people they are synonymous. Indeed, within the UK health service the assumption seems to be that the purpose of health promotion is primarily to influence healthy lifestyles by means of education. For instance, while it may not be absolutely clear what happens in so-called health promotion clinics in primary care, it is probable that the 'preventive medical model' of health education is alive and well. In short, patients are to be persuaded to submit themselves for screening and to adopt behaviours which are conducive to achieving the objectives of the *Health of the Nation*. There is indeed an element of novelty in this most recent specification for health education in general practice – the consultation is now no longer viewed as the prime locus for delivering the education, and practice nurses may be expected to take on the demanding role of running group education sessions (see Chapter 2 by Sturt for a deeper analysis of health promotion in general practice).

There is nothing fundamentally wrong with this prescription for health promotion in primary care. Indeed, it might be said that the aspirations of health educators in the early 1970s and the Royal College of General Practitioners in the early 1980s have at last been achieved. However, these activities are not health promotion as defined above. Although health education has a major part to play, health promotion is a much broader set of activities, and Figure 3.1 below demonstrates the nature of this educational contribution.

Over the years, several different models of health education have been described. These have been essentially ideological models, i.e. they assert what the purpose of health education ought to be, and advocates of one or other model challenge those who appear to favour an alternative approach. For instance, the traditional preventive model – which we suggested was the basis of most practice in health promotion clinics – derives its ideological thrust from the not unreasonable belief that it is a good idea to prevent disease. It also tends to carry with it certain non-essential baggage in the form of a 'medicalized' authoritarian view of the proper relationship between medical practitioner and client/patient. This relationship is nicely embodied in the term 'compliance' – which is supposedly a quality which patients should demonstrate in the face of medical advice. The well-established fact that some 50 per cent of patients fail to do so (e.g. Ley, 1990; Tones, 1997) seems to indicate a fundamental flaw in this particular aspect of the model! Clearly, however, while health promotion might applaud preventive goals, the authoritarian dimension associated with a medical model is anathema, since it is completely inconsistent with the overriding commitment to empowerment. Indeed, the goal of demedicalization, i.e. to diminish the power of medicine and its territorial claims, is part and parcel of WHO ideology together with its stated aim to 'reorient services'.

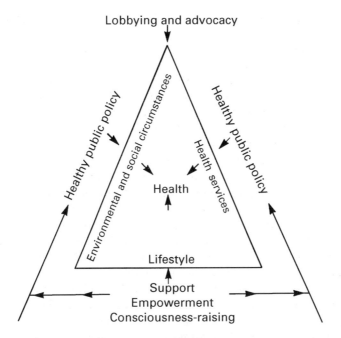

Figure 3.1 The contribution of education to health promotion

A radical option: healthy public policy

A health education model which subscribes to a substantially different philosophy from that espoused by the preventive model challenges the individual focus of traditional preventive approaches. To advocate individual lifestyle change is to 'blame the victims' of the social and environmental factors which create the unhealthy circumstances in the first place. Accordingly, a more radical approach is envisaged which seeks to bring about social and political change in order to make the healthy choice a more viable option (and doubtless to replace a dominant right-wing ideology with a more congenial radical alternative).

The radical option is fully compatible with the Ottawa Charter, which brought the matter of health policy to centre-stage and argued that there would be a global improvement in health only when governments made serious attempts to deal with the environmental and social circumstances which militated against health and nurtured disease. 'Political will' was needed in order to 'build healthy public policy' which would, in turn, generate legislation, create fiscal and economic circumstances, and literally engineer the environment to foster healthy living.

One subgoal of the policy-building process involved reorienting health services. This was not merely concerned with making medical services more accessible and user-friendly – by, for example, improving appointments systems and empowering patients. Rather it sought to broaden the way in which health services were conceptualized. Health services are not synonymous with medical services, and a whole variety of agencies and institutions can influence health positively or negatively. Good housing is of paramount importance for health; transport policy can be health-promoting; economic development corporations can foster health initiatives or stifle them. It is interesting to note not only the emphasis which the Ottawa Charter placed on building healthy public policy, but also the relatively minor role accorded to health education. The favoured method of influence was rather blandly described in terms of lobbying, 'mediation' and 'advocacy'. Obviously, lobbying is important and has always been associated with attempts to influence policy and the decision-making processes of government or other organizations and agencies. However, in the author's view, the apparent marginalization of health education in the Ottawa Charter was a fundamental error – doubtless deriving from a narrow preventive medical model view of health education's role and functions. As may be seen from Figure 3.1, health education operates in a kind of partnership with policy development. Its role is twofold. First of all, it seeks to influence individual lifestyle – but not in the traditional way. Its main purpose is not to coerce, cajole or persuade, but rather to facilitate choice by providing people with empowering competences and support. This empowering function also extends to the utilization of health services by helping patients to interact assertively with practitioners.

The second and perhaps more challenging function for health education is about community rather than individual empowerment. Its rationale is simple – lobbying and advocacy alone will not materially influence policies which benefit powerful individuals and corporate interests. Accordingly, vigorous public pressure and even the ballot box are prerequisites for substantial social changes. The underlying principles for this 'radical' approach have been established for some time, and can be encapsulated in Freire's (1974) term 'critical consciousness-raising' (CCR). A discussion of the philosophy and techniques of this approach is beyond the scope of this chapter, but may be found in Chapter 2 by Sturt. Suffice it to say that the purpose of CCR is to create a level of indignant awareness and concern in the public about factors militating against health. However, CCR must, be supported by the technology of empowerment if indignation is to be translated into community action.

At the very simplest level, the important symbiotic relationship between policy and education can be encapsulated in the following 'formula':

Health promotion = Health education x Healthy public policy.

Three common questions

Having spent some time reviewing the various contributions which health education might make to the achievement of the goals of health promotion, it will be useful at this point to remind ourselves of three rhetorical questions which are frequently posed by critics.

- Does it work ?
- What is it/should it be trying to do?
- Is it ethical ?

It is true that the order of these questions is not logical, but then, the underlying reason for asking the questions is not always logical. For instance, the question of effectiveness is often raised in the absence of any clear conceptualization of the nature and purpose of health education. Alternatively, the questioner may have a quite clear idea (often incorrect) of what health educators are trying to do. In this latter case, there may be a hidden agenda and – to use a term from linguistics – the three questions have a special illocutionary force. The three questions really mean: (i) health education does not work; (ii) it is trying to change people's lifestyle and behaviour; (iii) it is unethical, since it represents the attempts of sundry 'do-gooders' to spoil my pleasures and limit *my* freedom. In fact it is doubly unethical since it challenges my ideological world view and vision of what is right and wrong.

The question of effectiveness will receive some further consideration later in this chapter. However, we should note here that the health promotion formula presented above is highly relevant to the question of effectiveness. It asserts that without supportive public policy, health education will find success hard to achieve on a grand scale – just as policy goals will be difficult to achieve without education. As for the purposes of health education, these have been quite thoroughly explored above. Moreover, the standpoint adopted in this chapter may be stated unequivocally as being congruent with that of the WHO. Health education seeks to address the problem of inequalities in health. It seeks to create concern for others' rights to be healthy. It aims to give people a fairer share of power and to provide individuals with the competences and support they need to make health choices. Its purposes are thus fundamentally democratic – a point of especial significance when we consider the third of the questions listed above – is health education ethical ? We shall now give some consideration to that issue.

Ethics and the question of voluntarism

There are sufficient ethical issues in health education to justify the Society of Public Health Educators (SOPHE) of America establishing its own code of ethics (Faden and Faden, 1978). For instance, we must accept the possibility of an educational equivalent of iatrogenesis and, following the medical precept *'primum non nocere'*, at least expect health education to do no harm. Consequently, we would argue that it is not ethical to run mass media campaigns without routinely pre-testing messages in order to minimize the likelihood of unwanted side-effects – such as confusion or unproductive levels of fear or anxiety. Other instances might be provided, but further discussion of ethical matters will be limited to the accusation that health education and health promotion generally both have an unwarranted tendency to seek to restrict individual freedom and 'coerce' people into healthy activity.

Of course since health education, unlike medicine, is undertaken by a wide range of practitioners – both skilled and unskilled – it is not possible to make generalizations about the nature and extent of ethical or unethical practice. However, we should observe that the American professional body to which reference was made above (SOPHE) unequivocally affirmed in 1976 the importance of voluntarism in the following words:

> Health educators value privacy, dignity and the worth of the individual, and use skills consistent with these values. Health educators observe the principle of informed consent with respect to individuals and groups served. Health educators support change by choice, not by coercion.
>
> (Society of Public Health Educators, 1976)

However, it is ingenuous in the extreme to assume that people normally have anything approaching complete freedom of choice – or indeed that such a state is desirable. Before considering the extent to which health education can actually facilitate choice in accordance with SOPHE principles, let us acknowledge the existence of important impediments to action.

Barriers to choice

There are two significant barriers to individual freedom of choice. The first of these is by now familiar, and comprises those various environmental factors which are the preserve of healthy public policy. The second kind of barrier is better described as psychological, and operates in an often less obvious and more subtle way. However, in relation to the environmental barrier we must reiterate the observation that those reared and living in disadvantaged circumstances have their freedom of choice curtailed in a wide variety of ways. Indeed, it was for this reason that the first of the WHO's 38 targets for achieving HFA 2000 (World Health Organization, 1985) had as its objective that, by the year 2000, 'the actual differences in health status between countries and between groups within countries should be reduced by at least 25%, by improving the level of health of disadvantaged nations and groups.'

A more recent expression of concern about the social and environmental determinants of ill health and the associated barriers to choice has been made by the WHO ('Adolescent girls face a dangerous crossroads in life, says

WHO.' Press release, 3 October 1994). The following observation is made about the problems faced by many adolescent girls world-wide.

> Adolescence is one of life's most dangerous crossroads. Before they reach adulthood, their relative powerlessness and emerging sexuality leave them vulnerable to exploitation by others, and at risk of many forms of discrimination, violence, and ill health. Their health is jeopardized because often they have a low status in their families and in their workplaces, and crucially, fewer opportunities for education, training and employment. In such an atmosphere, they face hazards such as child marriage, child prostitution, genital mutilation, assault during pregnancy, courtship or dating violence, and sexual harassment and abuse.
>
> (World Health Organization, 1994)

We might legitimately ask what kind of freedom of choice adolescent girls enjoy in the circumstances outlined above!

At the individual psychological level, it is also apparent that complete freedom of choice is a relatively rare commodity and unequally distributed. Apart from lack of information, there may be many factors militating against people's capacity to choose freely. Those who are 'addicted' to some substance or other are not as free to choose to indulge in their habit as they were prior to their habituation – a fact that is amply illustrated by the very high proportion of smokers who claim that they would rather not be smoking. Again, there is consistent evidence that many people both know what is involved in healthy lifestyles and are motivated to improve their health status. What they lack is in part the skills and support needed to do so, and in part the belief that they are actually capable of exercising any influence over often debilitating social circumstances. Accordingly, it is either extremely cynical or extraordinarily naïve to pronounce that health education should not interfere in other people's lives and leave them either to choose their own pathway to health or to elect for a short but gratifying life! It is almost equally ingenuous to give the impression that only health educators are inclined to interfere with people's liberty.

Justification for coercion: utilitarianism and paternalism

We can envisage two kinds of coercion. The first is environmental, while the second represents what might be called 'psychological' coercion. Within the context of health promotion, various policy initiatives would seek to engineer changes in the environment while certain (so-called) educational measures might contribute to psychological change. Figure 3.2 represents these two dimensions in the form of a 'coercion continuum'.

At one end of the environmental spectrum is a kind of free-market *laissez-faire* approach, whilst the other pole represents substantial legislative, fiscal, economic and environmental interference.

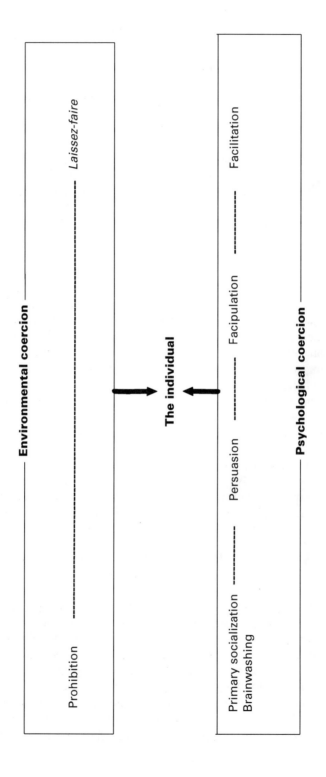

Figure 3.2 A coercion continuum

In health terms the left-hand pole would ensure that the healthy choice was the only possible choice! The spectrum of psychological coercion equally shows a range of interventions. To the left of the continuum (arguably) more powerful techniques are shown; at any rate, if their power can be doubted then their coercive intention cannot. Anti-interventionists might note, incidentally, that the most powerful and pervasive method of coercion is the cluster of strategies employed in rearing our children during the formative process of primary socialization! On the other hand, ethically appropriate empowerment techniques are shown at the right-hand side of the diagram. By way of further explanation, the term 'persuasion' would include the non-rational techniques liberally used by the advertising industry in manipulating choices of product – healthy or unhealthy. 'Facipulation' is a term coined by Constantino-David (1982) to describe a subtly manipulative tactic which might be used in community development (or certain counselling situations). While apparently facilitating the achievement of 'felt needs', the community worker or counsellor delicately suggests courses of action which meet the worker's own political or health agenda, but which leave clients convinced that they had thought of the idea in the first place.

Now the preferred position on the coercion continuum both for those who rally against interference by the 'nanny state' and for those ethically concerned health educators who seek to preserve the principle of volun-taristic choice is on the right (topographically speaking). Yet in many instances such a position is untenable. In brief, the adoption of coercive measures has been justified for many centuries in terms of utilitarianism and paternalism.

Only a limited discussion of these issues is possible here. Suffice it to say that the principle of utilitarianism states that people's freedom of action should be respected so long as it does not interfere with the general good. John Stuart Mill (1961) put it thus, 'The only purpose for which power can be rightfully exercised over any member of a civilised community, against his will, is to prevent harm to others. His own good, either physical or moral, is not sufficent warrant.' In fact there is a surprisingly large number of instances where power is exercised in order to prevent harm to others – or at any rate to the public purse. Health promotion is by no means unique in seeking to use healthy public policy to avoid damage to individuals and communities.

Although it might be arguable that power should not be exercised over others for their own good on utilitarian grounds, the principle of paternalism legitimizes this interference in certain cases. In short, we may coerce others who are deemed to be incapable for whatever reason of making rational decisions themselves. Ignorance may not be such a justification, but what about powerlessness or addiction? Maybe not, but being young has commonly been viewed as good grounds for having decisions made on one's behalf. Interestingly, LeFanu (1994) commented that health education appeared to be 'qualitatively different from most other forms of education whose aim is to impart knowledge or intellectual skills.' It is undoubtedly true that educational philosophers such as Hirst (1969) considered rationality to be the true purpose of education, but it would be widely accepted that this principle is rarely applied in educational practice. Certainly to choose schools as an example of 'pure' education is unwise, since by the very choice of curriculum, certain values are often quite pointedly applied. For instance, school pupils are obliged to spend some 15 000 hours being exposed to the UK National Curriculum. Politicians seeking to influence that curriculum in recent years have by no means been motivated to foster voluntaristic decision-making. Rather, the ideological drive has been to 'get back to basics' – which, in part, means to learn by rote rather than acquire decision-making skills. Moreover, a second quite blatant ideological thrust has been to try to convert the curriculum into a device to engender a rather narrow notion of 'enterprise' and to foster certain equally narrow 'family values'.

Again, with regard to the application of the principles of utilitarianism and paternalism, the philosophical stance of health promotion and the associated model of health education adopted here is certainly not anti-interventionist, but it is quite clearly voluntaristic. In short, it seeks to maximize the opportunities for communities and individuals to choose freely within the constraints imposed by concern for others' rights to do likewise. It aims to achieve these goals by using health policy to remove barriers to choice and education to empower decision-making.

These rather stirring statements of intent might reasonably bring accusations of empty rhetoric. However, contrary to some opinion, health education has a substantial corpus of theoretical wisdom with which to translate the rhetoric of empowerment into reality, and an attempt will now be made to provide some insight into this process.

A theory and technology of empowerment

So far, our references to health education have tended to be of an ideological nature, i.e. they have centred on its overriding purpose in terms of professional or moral values. We shall now give some consideration to what might best be termed the 'technological' aspects, i.e. the technical details involved in translating any given ideology into practice. In this respect, a definition of health education is not hard to formulate. It is conceptualized in this chapter as follows:

> Health education is any intentional activity which is designed to achieve health- or illness-related learning, i.e. some relatively permanent change in an individual's capability or disposition. Effective health education may therefore produce changes in knowledge and understanding or ways of thinking. It may influence or clarify values; it may bring about some shift in belief or attitude; it may facilitate the acquisition of skills; it may even effect changes in behaviour or lifestyle.

Although this definition is doubtless unsurprising to those who are professionally skilled, there still exists in those who are not an often remarkably naïve conception of what is involved in influencing people's health-related behaviours. There are still those who appear to believe that unhealthy lifestyles are due to ignorance, and who are consequently thoroughly surprised when individuals persist in their irresponsible ways despite having been provided with large quantities of information! Other self-styled experts will acknowledge the limitations of this simplistic notion that knowledge leads to practice (K——→P) and insert an 'A' into the 'formula' (K——→A——→P), arguing that attitudes must be changed before healthy practices can be adopted. Frequently the result of such an analysis is a mass media message containing simplistic information in a form designed to change attitudes (perhaps by a measured dose of fear appeal). If they have the courage to evaluate the success of the initiative, they are highly likely to record failure. Others will then confidently report yet another example of the ineffectiveness of health education.

Ironically, health education has a rich and sophisticated theoretical base on which to draw. The fact that this is often ignored by non-specialists is of some interest in its own right. It doubtless represents a lamentable tendency to assume that education is a quite simple and common-sense process – a point of great irritation to the teaching profession for very many years! Moreover, since health education has had a more or less close relationship with the medical profession over the years, it might also have something to do with the imbalance between the relative power and status of education and medicine!

Be that as it may, although there is a range of different social and behavioural science models and theories on which to draw, we do have a good understanding of what influences people's behaviours in health and illness – an observation which we shall now seek to illustrate.

Making health-related decisions

Many of the factors that influence individual decision-making are incorporated in the definition of health education provided earlier – explicitly or implicitly. Let us, for instance, consider what might influence a hypothetical individual's decision to respond to an educational interaction which is concerned with prudent use of drugs. It is doubtless clear that some knowledge and understanding of the nature and effects of the given substance would be necessary – people would need to understand about units of alcohol and the recommended healthy limits for consumption. Although necessary, such knowledge would not be sufficient. In addition, the individual in question would have to believe this 'healthy message', and might also need a number of supportive skills. He or she would undoubtedly benefit from social interaction skills training in order to resist pressure from peers in a 'round-buying culture' to have unwanted drinks.

First aid skills would also be useful for occasions when friends may have overdosed!

The importance of people's beliefs in the decision-making process cannot be overestimated. Indeed, ensuring that individuals' health-related beliefs correspond to current realities might well be the main concern of the educational endeavour. For instance, the celebrated Health Belief Model (e.g. Janz and Becker, 1984) offers useful guidance for those seeking to persuade clients to adopt safer sex practices. For example, before condom use becomes a more attractive proposition, clients must be reasonably convinced that they are susceptible to HIV infection, they must believe that the outcome of infection will be serious, they must accept that condoms are actually beneficial in acting as a barrier to the virus, and they need to balance this (and any other) perceived benefit against the costs which they might believe condom use will incur.

Although useful, the Health Belief Model (HBM) has its limitations. For instance, we must certainly reckon with another category of belief in addition to those highlighted by the HBM. We must take into account people's beliefs about the nature and cause of diseases (sometimes described in terms of attributions of causality). The relevance of this theoretical construct is well illustrated by the many reviews of myths about cancers. If, for instance, people believe that cancer is a single undifferentiated disease or that it lies dormant within each person as a seed, only waiting for one of many 'triggers' to generate overt disease, then it is hardly surprising that pessimism about treatment and prevention prevails, and delay in seeking medical help is not uncommon. Accordingly, health educators need to acknowledge these various 'theories of illness'. Indeed, Tuckett *et al.* (1985) argued that the exploration of patients' concepts and beliefs about their condition should be a *sine qua non* of effective medical consultations.

Any respectable theory must, of course, take account of people's motivational state. For instance, decisions about sexual practices will inevitably be influenced by individual value systems. As would be expected, moral values will be particularly relevant but paradoxically may prove a handicap unless they are sufficiently powerful that they enable individuals to 'resist temptation'. The worst possible scenario is where, say, a moral imperative prevents a young woman even contemplating anticipatory purchase of a condom, but is not quite strong enough to prevent her yielding to the power of the sex drive!

Further consideration of the HBM's central concept of perceived susceptibility requires more sophisticated analysis. It is self-evident that some people are actually motivated by a belief in susceptibility to certain kinds of risk. They may be 'sensation-seekers'; they may enjoy the experience of maintaining control 'at the edge' (Lyng, 1990). At all events they will not co-operate with health education messages emphasizing the risk of damage to their health. Indeed, one of the more revealing conceptualizations of the reasons why adolescents frequently engage in health-threatening behaviours is embodied in Jessor and Jessor's (1977) theory of problem behaviour. In short, health-compromising activities (such as delinquent or antisocial behaviour) are symptomatic. Accordingly, health promotion must again address root causes – a point we shall revisit when we later note the disadvantages of 'vertical' programmes.

All we can hope to do here is to provide a vignette which supports our earlier assertion that we have a rich theoretical tapestry at our disposal if we care to use it to explain individuals' decision-making processes in health and illness. However, even a brief review must give some consideration to those psychosocial and environmental factors which contribute directly to the empowerment of decisions. This we shall now attempt to provide.

The dynamics of empowerment

The concept of empowerment is central to the philosophy and practice of health promotion. In one sense it parallels the concept of health – it can be said to be both a desirable end in itself and a means to an end. So, just as the WHO has come to regard health as a means of achieving a socially and economically productive life, empowerment of individuals and communities acts instrumentally to facilitate 'healthy' decision-making.

The concept of empowerment is both complex and 'slippery', and only some of its bare bones can be mentioned here (for a more complete review, see Tones, 1992; Tones and Tilford, 1994). In short, empowerment has to do with the relationship between individuals and their environment; the relationship is reciprocal. This reciprocity factor is central to Social Learning Theory, and Bandura (1982, 1986) has emphasized the importance of recognizing the phenomenon of 'reciprocal determinism'. Clearly the environment may exercise a powerful controlling influence on people, but people may also influence their environment. For instance, as a collective, a community might put pressure on authorities – local or national – in order to achieve change (see Figure 3.1). Communities might also take direct action to improve their environments. Again, individuals may exert pressure for change (perhaps after a process of critical consciousness-raising) by lobbying or through the ballot box.

At the micro-level, empowerment is also a key health promotion goal. For instance, as part of client contract behaviour modification, people might learn how to avoid environmental circumstances which trigger their consumption of tobacco or alcohol, they might acquire skills in resisting social pressure, and they might learn how to control 'temptation' by applying self-regulatory skills and by rewarding themselves with some substitute gratifications. As we shall note later, such techniques need to be incorporated into many health promotion consultations – either face to face or within a group context. They also provide a clear example of how the rhetoric of empowerment can be operationalized and translated into specific educational objectives.

As should be evident from the preceding discussion, these empowering tactics draw on a corpus of sophisticated research and psychological constructs. A comprehensive account is not possible here, but key self-empowerment concepts include beliefs about control (e.g. perceived locus of control and self-efficacy beliefs), values such as self-esteem and a variety of specific social and personal skills which might be encapsulated in the terms 'health and life skills'. Some of these are shown in Figure 3.3 below.

Figure 3.3 may be interpreted in the light of early observations about the limitations of the ' K——→A——→P' formula. First, the provision of knowledge must be supplemented by a process of values clarification in order to facilitate decision-making. Second, and in order to fulfil the criteria of empowerment, mere knowledge must be accompanied by the state of heightened and critical awareness which is the goal of critical consciousness-raising.

This 'superior brand' of knowledge is none the less not sufficient to influence intention and attitude in a satisfactory health-promoting fashion.

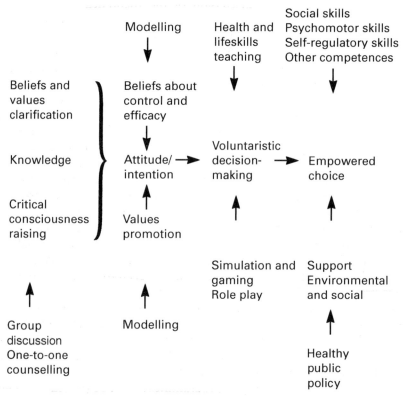

Figure 3.3 An empowerment model of health education

Individuals must also believe that they are capable of achieving what they would like to achieve – in short, they will need to acquire self-efficacy beliefs. We should also note that the educational process is not value free in the sense that any decision is acceptable so long as it is empowered! Figure 3.3 emphasizes the need for active 'values promotion'; for example, decisions should be 'responsible'. Although responsibility frequently seems to mean behaving in accordance with the often rather narrow moral principles espoused by the communicator, its definition here is quite broad. The moral imperative is essentially voluntaristic and utilitarian. The guideline is that people's decisions are ethical provided that they do not harm others and do not impinge on others' freedom to act.

Figure 3.3 also incorporates the central requirement of a supportive environment. Apart from demonstrating the need to provide supportive health and life skills – as mentioned above – it asserts the principle that healthy public policy is necessary to ensure that the healthy choice is the easy choice (but not the only choice!).

The importance of horizontal programmes

The preceding rather brief discussion of the theoretical basis of health education has hopefully provided some insight into the complex network of psychological, social and environmental factors which influence the adoption and maintenance of health-related behaviours. The importance of the synergistic relationship between education and health and social policy has also been stated. All of these factors lead to an inescapable conclusion – a narrow focus on the prevention of specific diseases is not necessarily the most effective and certainly not the most economical way of tackling the health problems in question. Although not logically inevitable, the specification of five 'key areas' for action in the *Health of the Nation* will very probably lead to thinking in terms of 'vertical' programmes, i.e. programmes focused on a single disease or set of behaviours. By contrast, recognition that specific outcomes are usually the result of a complex of many underlying influences should lead to the adoption of 'horizontal' programmes (Tones, 1993a). Figure 3.4 is probably self-explanatory, but we might none the less note that healthy public policy designed to ameliorate the social conditions which militate against healthy choices is shown as the foundation of a horizontal approach. The phenomenon of reciprocal determinism is demonstrated in the interaction of policy with the next 'layer' of health and lifeskills. Both influence lifestyle, i.e. the range of behaviours traditionally targeted by health education. However, even at the level of lifestyle, it is well recognized that the same lifestyle factor, such as diet, may contribute to the risk of a number of specific diseases, including two of the five areas chosen for priority action in the *Health of the Nation*.

The ease with which horizontal programmes might be provided depends substantially on context and setting. The so-called 'settings approach' has

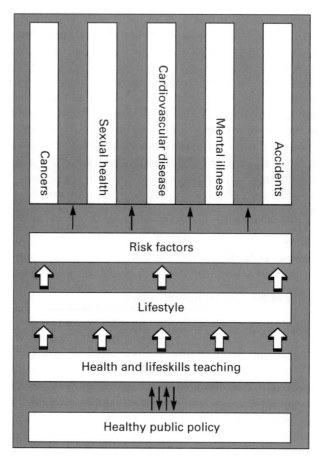

Figure 3.4 Contribution of horizontal programmes

received a great deal of attention in recent years and will also receive some quite brief consideration here.

Methods and strategies: settings and contexts

Although there is no universal agreement about defining the main terms to be discussed below, we are using the expressions 'setting' and 'context' virtually interchangeably. 'Setting' does tend to suggest a deliberate decision to deliver a programme, whereas 'context' can be used to acknowledge the fact that a need for health promotion might arise, e.g. as part of a community development initiative. 'Strategy', on the other hand, involves a broader planning process – perhaps to use mass media or to develop an integrated CHD prevention programme. The term 'method' is best used to describe activities at the micro-level, e.g. the use of specific techniques such as those shown in Figure 3.3 above, namely group discussion, counselling, use of role play and deliberate use of models to influence beliefs or demonstrate skills.

Settings and contexts

Matters to do with methods, strategies and settings have been more fully explored elsewhere (Bracht, 1990; Whitehead and Tones, 1990; Tones, 1993b). We shall therefore merely make a number of observations here and emphasize a few principles.

First, and obviously, there is a wide variety of possible settings in which health promotion might be provided – schools, primary medical care, hospitals and the workplace are among the most popular. Each of these provides a particular ethos and has its own peculiar strengths and limitations. For instance, schools have a more or less captive audience; young people spend some 15 000 hours at a relatively formative stage in their health careers in the ambit of schools. Moreover, schoolteachers have a good deal of credibility together with a wide range of methodological skills. Again, of particular importance in the light of our earlier observation, the school can and sometimes does implement a full horizontal programme as part of its personal, social and health education programme. Moreover, the school was the first setting to recognize the complementarity of education and policy. This happened initially when health educationists acknowledged the importance of the 'hidden curriculum' in complementing or, alternatively, contradicting the school's teaching activities. More recently, this synergy between teaching and policy has been 'legitimized' in the form of a 'health-promoting school' network in Europe (Nutbeam *et al.*, 1991). On the other hand, there are limitations to what the school can achieve. For instance, 'delinquescent' groups of students may routinely react against what they perceive as imposed authority. Again, innumerable demands are made on curriculum time, and health promotion may appear relatively low on the priority list for some school governors and teachers; accordingly, many topics may receive unbalanced or sketchy treatment. At all events the importance of the school as part of an integrated community-wide programme of health promotion cannot be exaggerated.

As with schools, other agencies, institutions and settings can make their own special contributions. It is sufficient here to comment on only one more of these – the hospital sector.

The notion of a health-promoting hospital is interesting in the present context for many reasons. First, many people would have considered that the hospital would be the last place in which the principles of health promotion might be applied! The fact is that, following the Budapest Declaration (World Health Organization, 1991), strenuous and deliberate efforts have been made in certain quarters to create a model health promotion setting. The historical antecedents of this development will not receive further elaboration; we shall merely note that the initiative followed logically from the Healthy Cities and Health-Promoting Schools movements, and record the following main principles which those aspiring to the status of Health-Promoting Hospital must follow.

- There should be a focus on health rather than on disease.
- The environment should be conducive to health promotion – there should not only be complementary health policies (e.g. nutrition and smoking), but the hospital should also set a good example to other workplaces by having a model occupational health service catering for the needs of all its staff.
- Extending (quite considerably) the notion of a patient's charter, patients and their relatives should be the beneficiaries of good communication and sound health education.
- There should be a concerted effort to actively empower patients *and staff* (my emphasis).
- The hospital should have an epidemiological database. It should be outward-looking, seek support from voluntary bodies and establish a 'healthy alliance' with the community which it serves.

It will be obvious that at least three of the WHO's major concerns are incorporated prominently in the above list, namely healthy public policy, empowerment and intersectoral collaboration. Moreover, the UK Department of Health has provided some degree of legitimacy to the venture in a recent publication (Department of Health, 1994).

Following the numerous references made to equity and empowerment, we cannot leave our discussion of settings, strategies and contexts without commenting, however briefly, on what for many people is the empowerment strategy *par excellence* – community development (CD). The rationale and ideology of this grass roots movement can be stated quite simply. Its fundamental purpose is to remedy inequitable distribution of power and resources. It works with communities (i.e. relatively small geographical entities having common circumstances or goals together with an extended network of interpersonal contacts) and does so in an informal manner. It helps communities to identify their 'felt needs', seeks to raise their consciousness about social circumstances, and aims to facilitate change by means of community participation and empowerment. It is therefore quite different in intent from other 'outreach' programmes which, by contrast, work in a 'top-down' fashion and seek, as it were, to 'colonize' disadvantaged communities and 'get the message through' to the 'hard to reach'. Outreach strategies of this latter type, while apparently conforming to the requirements of community development, may actually be depowering in their imposition of a preventive medical agenda. In relation to our earlier discussion of voluntarism and coercion, the skilful infiltration of community networks without taking account of community felt needs is a good example of 'facipulation'.

Again, the strategic use of the mass media must be considered in any review of community-wide health promotion activities. This subject has been discussed elsewhere and cannot receive detailed treatment here. A more complete review may be found in Tones and Tilford (1994) and Backer *et al.* (1992). However, we might at some risk of superficiality, summarize the contribution which the mass media might be expected to make to a community-wide programme in the following way.

- Mass media campaigns can be very successful at agenda-setting and critical consciousness-raising – provided that sufficient resources are devoted to achieving proper audience coverage.
- Mass media campaigns are least effective in changing beliefs, attitudes and behaviours – especially where such change involves significant loss of gratification or entails discomfort.
- The incidental effects of the mass media may be substantial – in the form of soap opera, for instance, they can raise awareness of issues, reinforce prejudice and put into cliché form the values and beliefs of their audience. One of the more important policy concerns of health promotion is therefore to influence media and publicity decision-making.
- Probably the most cost-effective way of utilizing the mass media is by means of unpaid media publicity.
- The mass media are most effective when supported by and supportive of interpersonal education provided in the various settings and contexts discussed above.

Frequent references have been made above to 'community-wide' programmes. We shall therefore complete this review of settings by reiterating a truism. The effectiveness of health promotion – as judged by evaluation at a macro-level – will be considerably enhanced by collaboration between all settings and by supportive public policy. Where all institutions and agencies subscribe to the same goals and provide similar messages, success is more probable. Where they utilize their peculiar advantages – of contact with client groups and of credibility, etc. – objectives will be more efficiently achieved. In fact, increasing interest is being shown in the American concept of 'community coalitions'. Apart from the benefits of healthy alliances between agencies and settings, it is argued that the active support of the great, the good and the powerful will enhance the prospect of success (Goodman *et al.*, 1993).

Health promotion at the micro-level

As we noted earlier, specific methods designed to promote efficient learning will operate within the various contexts and settings mentioned above.

Group discussion and assertiveness training, for example, might be observed in schools, the workplace or the community. It is at what we have called the micro-level that the grand principles of health promotion and empowerment must be converted into actual specific operations. Clearly, certain settings are more appropriate than others for encouraging particular kinds of learning.

For instance, raising critical consciousness about social issues might be more readily achieved within a personal and social education course for young people aged 16–19 years than in the health-promoting hospital. On the other hand, each setting can make a contribution and, as we noted in the preceding section, these contributions may be complementary and cumulative if they form part of a coherent community-wide strategy.

Primary care undoubtedly provides one of the most important contexts for health promotion, whether it be in the form of group work with patients or the more familiar one-to-one encounter between doctor or nurse and patient. Accordingly, we shall now identify some of the potential ways in which the health practitioner can contribute to client empowerment as part of this face-to-face educational (and possibly therapeutic) interaction. The major features of this educational interaction are summarized in Figure 3.5.

For the sake of simplicity, the practitioner–client interaction is shown in Figure 3.5 as a one-way process, with the practitioner seeking to communicate with clients, motivate them and provide them with post-decisional support. In reality, of course, the process is a two-way one. For instance, in order to check beliefs or gain insight into his or her environmental circumstances, there must be full client participation. Indeed, this high level of involvement is at the heart of the empowerment process. Moreover, the educational encounter should be a significant learning experience for the educator; the doctor or nurse should gain valuable insights, e.g. into the social circumstances which militate against patient co-operation with advice.

Communication is here conceptualized as the process of transmitting information to clients in an intelligible fashion. The client's task is to 'decode' the message by paying attention and correctly interpreting the message. In order to achieve satisfactory communication, the communicator must seek continuing feedback from the client to ensure that correct interpretation and understanding have been achieved. This should, of course, be part of practitioners' skills – along with a capacity to manage non-verbal communication (NVC) and to deliver the message in a form which is matched to the learning readiness of the client.

Clearly, the purpose of most consultations in primary care is not merely to ensure that patients correctly interpret the information presented to them. More commonly, the concern of the doctor or nurse is to influence behaviour. Accordingly, in addition to communication, Figure 3.5 shows two further stages in the educational process. The focus of the second stage is on motivation. However, following the dictates of health promotion, the purpose of the interaction with the patient is not passive compliance with

EDUCATION TASK **CLIENT TASK**

Communication
Check felt needs/need for information
Establish rapport using counselling skills, active listening, etc; take account of NVC
Check for understanding
Check intelligibility of written information
Take steps to maximize recall/provide *aide-mémoire* if necessary

Receive message: pay attention
Perceive and interpret message correctly

Motivation: facilitating decision-making

Explore existing beliefs, attitudes, skills
Seek to modify beliefs and attitudes where appropriate
Provide information; provide skills: decision-making psychomotor, social and lifeskills
Check learning and recall
Analyse environmental circumstances
Negotiate and agree 'contract'

Form appropriate beliefs (e.g. about causes and nature of disease and health issues, about susceptibility, seriousness, costs and benefits of recommended actions)

Develop self-efficacy benefits
Acquire skills
Agree contract

Provide support
Provide opportunity for acquiring supportive knowledge, social and self-regulatory skills
Help to mobilize social and environmental support
Act as advocate for social and environmental change
Check client's progress

Positive attitude/intention to act

Acquire new information and skills

Adopt and sustain health action

Improved health

Figure 3.5 The educational task

'doctor's orders', nor even the application of high-pressure persuasion to choose health, but rather the facilitation of choice. Part of this process involves taking account of the psychosocial and environmental factors which influence health- and illness-related behaviours, as discussed earlier in this chapter. Consequently, the motivational task involves working with client beliefs, values and attitudes. It involves providing necessary knowledge and skills. It also involves a joint review of relevant environmental and social circumstances. The client's learning task operates in parallel with and in response to the practitioner's educational efforts. If clients are to learn and acquire a positive attitude to the adoption of new and healthy activities, they will often need to change their beliefs, acquire new skills, etc. Moreover, before this newly acquired learning can be translated into practice, it will typically be necessary to provide social and environmental support. In fact, the provision of support is an essential and characteristic feature of the empowerment process. However, before leaving this analysis of the educational encounter, let us note more explicitly those features of the interaction which, in addition to the marshalling of support, can be described as empowering.

First of all, and as noted above, the relationship between practitioner and patient is of paramount importance. The traditional imbalance of power between doctor and patient and the associated notion of the sick role are quite clearly inconsistent with client participation and empowerment. Indeed, the inconsistency between expecting patients to comply with medical advice and, at the same time, respond to exhortations to 'look after yourself' has been recognized for some time. Tuckett *et al.* (1985) drew our attention to the fact that a significant proportion of patients were 'not committed' to their doctors' recommendations (in part due to perceived environmental barriers, and in part due to the fact that they did not appear to believe the advice!). However, they very rarely felt able to raise their doubts or to express their disagreements. Consequently, Tuckett advised doctors first of all to explore patients' 'theories of illness', beliefs and general concerns. In order to do this and, at the same time, to remedy the possible imbalance of power between client and practitioners, doctors must have at their disposal a set of effective social interaction skills. In other words, they need to operate in accordance with the 'holy trinity' of counselling and to demonstrate 'respect, empathy and genuineness'. They need to know how to listen actively, ask appropriate 'open' questions, provide feedback of feelings and generally demonstrate the specific competences which are conducive to facilitating choice. It is a generally gratifying – and empowering – experience to be consulted, involved and respected. This observation is consistent with Macleod Clark's conceptualization of 'health nursing' rather than 'sick nursing' (Macleod Clark, 1993), and has practical implications for health promotion, including such problematic enterprises as facilitating smoking cessation (Macleod Clark *et al.*, 1990). Providing people with 'unconditional positive regard' enhances their self-esteem. In fact, the social skills described above should form the basis of a new, health-promoting 'bedside manner'. Furthermore, apart from the pleasure which practitioners will doubtless gain from experiencing patient satisfaction, the use of these 'demystified' counselling skills provides the best opportunity for them to acquire the information they need to make an accurate diagnosis. The diagnosis, incidentally, may be a diagnosis of illness or the educational and social diagnosis which is necessary to help patients to deal with problematic social circumstances and to empower their health choices.

More particularly, in the context of motivating healthy decisions, we may note three other important tasks in the health-promoting consultation. The first of these is to influence self-efficacy beliefs. Unless clients believe that they are capable of achieving a desired goal, they will take no action. In order to achieve this goal, the practitioner might choose to use an appropriate 'model' – a person similar in characteristics and circumstances to the client, but who has in fact managed to achieve change. Alternatively, or additionally, clients may need to be provided with actual competences and skills which make it possible for them to achieve success and, in this particular context, it is indeed true that nothing succeeds like success!

The second task is concerned with the detailed analysis of clients' circumstances. If social or environmental factors militate against individual choice, recommendations to make lifestyle changes will almost certainly be ineffective. Indeed, to seek to do so when environmental circumstances are particularly oppressive involves a degree of 'victim-blaming' and may well be unethical! On the other hand, if the environment seems to be conducive to change and the client is persuaded that change is possible, some form of agreement – formal or informal – would ideally be drawn up. This 'contract', which identifies both practitioner and client roles and commitments, will make clear what steps are necessary for change – and enhance motivation. This contracting phase thus constitutes an important empowering aspect of the motivational process.

Finally, and unsurprisingly, the active provision of support is necessary to 'make the healthy choice the easy choice'. At one level this is not difficult, and supportive information may be all that is needed. More usually, however, supportive skills will be required. These might include various 'health skills' needed to cope with social pressures, or 'self regulatory' skills. The latter refer to competences which are particularly necessary when clients are likely to find it difficult not only to make decisions about adopting healthier behaviours, but also to sustain them. The most common example is 'addiction' to various substances, in which the decision to quit is easier than sustaining that intention. Self-regulatory skills can assist with this process.

Creating change in the environment itself is, of course, much more problematic. While a practitioner might well be able to mobilize social support – an extremely powerful determinant of healthy-decision making – influencing the physical or socio-economic environment may just not be possible. Perhaps a doctor or social worker might manage to have a family rehoused or help with income support, but it would be naïve to expect such actions to have anything but a minimal effect on social ills such as poverty or unemployment and, of course, the feelings of helplessness and depowerment associated with these. It is clearly unreasonable to expect any individual health worker to take on such a responsibility. However, we should remember that the Ottawa Charter urged all health professionals and their professional bodies to act as lobbyists and advocates for healthy public policy! We should also note that healthy alliances and community coalitions might achieve more substantial change by co-operative action.

Success in health promotion: effectiveness and efficiency

Anything other than a partial view of the effectiveness of health promotion is beyond the scope of this chapter, and those who are interested in the ideology and technology of evaluation should see, for instance, Green and Lewis (1986), Sarvela and McDermott (1993) and Tones and Tilford (1994). None the less, bearing in mind the regular and often somewhat petulant demands that health promotion/health education should justify their existence, some observations are necessary at this juncture.

First of all, merely to ask whether health promotion works (or worse, to assert that it does not!) is to pose a rather meaningless question akin to asking whether health services are effective. However, it is legitimate to ask about the effectiveness and efficiency of particular health promotion endeavours, and we should remind ourselves about the meaning of these two terms. Effectiveness refers to the extent to which a programme achieves its goals. Efficiency refers to its relative effectiveness, i.e. how well it achieves its goals (or the standards and conditions built into its objectives) by comparison with alternative and competing approaches. Before we can address this matter we must, of course, ask about the goals themselves or, more precisely, the values embodied in those goals.

The purpose of evaluation is to measure success. Statements about success depend on goals and, as we have often noted, the criteria for success depend on the ideological basis of our programmes. Accordingly, before we can make any sensible observation about the effectiveness of health promotion, we need to be clear about this ideological basis. For instance, if we were to incorporate the broad aims of the Ottawa Charter into our programmes and use these as a basis for evaluation, we might look for evidence of having achieved greater equity. We might target William Beveridge's 'five giants of disease, idleness, ignorance, squalor and want' and judge our success by how many we have slain! It would, of course, be entirely unrealistic to use such broad outcomes as indicators of success, and we would need to identify appropriate and specific indicators of effectiveness.

More usually, however, the success of health promotion will not be assessed in terms of substantial social change or even empowerment *per se*, but rather in relation to the narrower aims of preventive medicine and, in the UK, by the extent to which the *Health of the Nation* targets have been met. Since we have argued here that an empowerment approach is also likely to achieve preventive outcomes, the rest of our discussion of effectiveness will relate to either the attainment of preventive goals or the state of empowerment which, arguably, facilitates the achievement of those preventive outcomes. However, this discussion will be prefaced by an assertion which may be a little controversial. It is that the success of health promotion and health education programmes should not be judged by traditional epidemiological indicators such as mortality and morbidity. Various intermediate and indirect indicators of effectiveness must be used, and their selection must be based on sound understanding of social and behavioural science.

The importance of intermediate indicators

The assertion made above may perhaps be a little surprising. After all, if health promotion is to achieve preventive outcomes, is it not reasonable to assess success in terms of reductions in mortality or morbidity? There are two main reasons for not doing so. First, there is frequently some degree of uncertainty associated with the postulated links between particular behaviours and specific disease outcomes, at any rate on a population basis. It is thus decidedly unreasonable to claim that health education has been ineffective if it has influenced lifestyle but this behaviour change has not (at least yet) manifested itself in a reduction in disease. It might, of course, be argued that the education in question is therefore not worthwhile without concrete proof of medical benefit. However, apart from the fact that such proof is inherently difficult to obtain, many behaviours have multiple benefits in that they might reduce risk factors for a number of particular conditions (as we demonstrated in our earlier discussion of the need for horizontal programmes). A second justification for looking for intermediate indicators is based on the logical observation that a particular educational input may not show any benefit at all for many years. For instance, successful cancer education in schools could not be expected to influence the adoption of mammography screening until the girls in question had achieved middle age!

Perhaps an even more important reason for using intermediate indicators derives from the fact that, as we have seen, individuals' decisions about health or illness are multiply determined. They do not follow a simple linear progression, e.g. from knowledge to attitude change to behaviour. One single 'input' – whether this be simple or complex – is therefore unlikely to achieve a desired 'output'. To measure effectiveness by looking for evidence of a successful output would normally be inappropriate. For instance, consider a hypothetical mass media programme which seeks to influence dietary practices. At the very least, the following chain of events would have to take place. The target audience would first need to be adequately exposed to the message and become aware of its existence. They would need to interpret it correctly and understand it. They would need to believe it and assess its personal relevance, and they would typically consider the possible costs and benefits involved in undertaking the dietary changes recommended by the programme and assess the likelihood of their having the expertise and stamina needed to make those changes. If these various steps have been successfully negotiated, and if the audience has not been antagonized or made anxious by the message, a positive attitude to adopting a healthy diet might emerge. Of course, before that attitude can be translated into practice, the client group will doubtless need a variety of skills, additional knowledge and, of course, they must be able to find the healthy products and be able to afford them. If we simplify the above process into a sequence of 'awareness-knowledge-beliefs-attitudes-support-action' and assign hypothetical probabilities of each stage being satisfactorily 'negotiated', then the likelihood of success might be depicted as follows:

AWARENESS – KNOWLEDGE – BELIEFS – ATTITUDES – SUPPORT – ACTION

$$80\% \quad x \quad 50\% \quad x \quad 40\% \quad x \quad 30\% \quad x \quad 50\% \quad = \quad 2.4\%$$

The 'equation' above is based on 80 per cent of the audience achieving prompted recall of the message, but only 50 per cent of those understanding and remembering it. Of that 50 per cent only 40 per cent actually believe it, and 30 per cent of that 40 per cent develop a positive attitude and intention to act. This intention does not materialize in 50% of these cases due to inadequate support. The net result is an overall success rate of 2.4 per cent.

In other words, in order to improve effectiveness, the mass media input would need to be complemented by a variety of different educational interventions. These would be designed to achieve different learning outcomes, and would be delivered over a period of time in a variety of contexts and settings. Ideally, the educational programme would be supplemented by appropriate healthy public policy. Accordingly, it makes sense to assess each of these inputs separately. For instance, understanding of the nutritional basis might best be provided in schools – and assessed there. Empowerment-related beliefs and attitudes could also be supplied in the personal and social education programme within the school and/or in community development work (perhaps in the context of a food co-operative). Supportive policy might be created by providing healthy options in the works canteen and food labelling in the supermarket. Evaluation would therefore centre on the development and implementation of these policies. Bearing in mind our knowledge of mass media potential, evaluation of this aspect of the overall programme would be restricted to concept testing, pre-testing and assessment of penetration and acceptability.

Hopefully the reason for making the earlier statement about the inappropriateness of using epidemiological indicators of effectiveness will now be clear. Indeed, it would seem that the use of behavioural indicators will often not be the most appropriate way to evaluate success. Accordingly, we must look for intermediate indicators such as the beliefs and skills which represent successful learning outcomes, and which contribute in the long term to healthy decision-making. In fact, the recommended processes involved in communicating, motivating and providing support which are presented in Figure 3.5 actually provide a number of possible intermediate outcome measures.

On some occasions, intermediate indicators may not be necessary and 'indirect' indicators may be all that is needed. For example, we may need to appraise the efficiency of a communication skills course provided for practice nurses. The assumption is that if the course is sound, the trainees will become more skilled in educating their clients. Their new skill will in turn ultimately be revealed in more effective work with patients. In the longer term they and the course they have completed may contribute to behaviour change – and even have some small impact on the prevalence of disease!

Evidence of success

We should acknowledge that there are relatively few evaluations of fully fledged, integrated and genuine health promotion programmes – for the obvious reason that these are decidedly thin on the ground! Indeed, for a variety of reasons, it is probably more worthwhile to use our grasp of theory to develop and evaluate specific small-scale endeavours, while at the strategic level seeking to achieve co-ordinated programmes, as discussed above. Having said this, it would be churlish not to acknowledge that very real successes have been documented. We shall conclude the chapter with a few selective citations.

First, let us note Warner's (1989) observation that (in a US context), 'In the absence of the antismoking campaign, adult *per capita* cigarette consumption in 1987 would have been an estimated 78–89% higher than the level actually experienced.' As a result, 'an estimated 789 200 Americans avoided or postponed smoking-related deaths and gained an average of 21 additional years of life expectancy each.'

Of course, we cannot prove that the very real effects described by Warner are due to health education alone; indeed, it is not possible in retrospect to ascribe any specific causes. However, by definition the effects must logically have been due to health promotion, i.e. a combination of policy and education.

By contrast, a school- and community-based health education programme in South Carolina demonstrated specific relationships between input and output. It showed rather conclusively that, compared with three comparison counties, statistically significant reductions occurred in adolescent pregnancy rates (Vincent *et al.*, 1987). According to the researchers, the target county showed a 'remarkably sustained decline ... not observed in comparison counties' whose unwanted pregnancy rate increased during the same period.

We have said that effectiveness relates to the achievement of programme goals, whereas efficiency describes the relative effectiveness of a programme (i.e. its efficiency) by comparison with alternative measures. Perhaps the most stringent measures of efficiency are those which are described in terms of financial costs and benefits. Health promotion can in fact provide some examples of success according to these more demanding requirements. For instance, recent analyses in the UK have demonstrated the efficiency of GPs providing advice to stop smoking in accordance with these quite stringent criteria. For a budget of £1 million, this relatively straightforward intervention notched up 5988 Quality Adjusted Life Years (QALYs) compared to a much lower figure for breast cancer screening (302 QALYs), and even for hip replacement. This latter surgical intervention costs £750 per QALY compared with £167 for smoking-related advice (Godfrey *et al.*, 1989).

However, although we do have evidence that health promotion can be cost-effective, it is dangerous to place too much emphasis on economic appraisal. While cost-effectiveness may be a sensible pursuit so long as it enables planners to select the cheaper of two equally effective courses of action, cost-benefit analysis – by comparison – is distinctly more problematic. Ultimately, the costs of many health procedures (in monetary terms) may not be outweighed by the benefits. Even allowing for 'discounting', really efficient health promotion (like really efficient therapy) will ultimately be costly. In the last analysis the only really efficient financial expedient is to ensure that people live a productive and disease-free life so long as they contribute to the economy and then, having reached retirement age, die as soon as possible thereafter!

Perhaps the most useful approach to this dilemma is to follow the recommendations made by Cohen (1981). Prevention should be treated as a 'merit good', i.e. something which satisfies a 'merit want'. Merit wants are, according to Musgrave – cited by Cohen (1981) 'so meritorious that their satisfaction is provided for through the public budget over and above what is provided for through the market and paid for by private buyers.'

Since emphasis has been given in this chapter to empowerment and to the need for intermediate indicators, we shall close with some very revealing qualitative research evidence on the impact of drama on a number of health outcomes (Durrant, 1993). The scenario is the somewhat unlikely context of general practice. A GP involved in a scheme which addressed health issues through drama provides a good example of effectiveness. He made the following observation about the effectiveness of the programme: 'We have seen people grow in confidence, make important decisions, get on better with their families, have more patience with their children, make friends, and grow as people'. A community health worker who participated in the same project provides an additional insight into the empowerment benefits gained by those patients who were involved in the drama:

> *As they gain confidence in the sessions, they take this out on to the street, and this is seen in their daily lives. They feel they can apply for jobs they thought they never could have applied for, move to better houses, take on the council about the poll tax or the water meters, or allowances. We have people here now who wouldn't think twice about making a banner and campaigning outside the Town Hall to save local amenities.*

In short, perhaps we should replace John Webster's celebrated dictum 'Seek Wisely to Prevent' with an exhortation to 'Seek Wisely to Empower'! Through empowerment we may achieve ideologically sound success while addressing the needs of preventive medicine. We have the theoretical framework and the technical competences to achieve both of these goals.

References

Backer, T.E., Rogers, E.M. and Sopory, P. 1992: *Designing health communication campaigns: what works?* Newbury Park, CA: Sage.

Bandura, A. 1982: Self-efficacy mechanism in human agency. *American Psychologist* **37**, 122–47.

Bandura, A. 1986: *Social foundations of thought and action: a social cognitive theory.* Englewood Cliffs, NJ: Prentice Hall.

Bracht, N. (ed.) 1990: *Health promotion at the community level.* London: Sage.

Cohen, D. 1981: *Prevention as an economic good.* Aberdeen: Health Economics Research Unit, University of Aberdeen.

Constantino-David, K. 1982: Issues in community organization. *Community Development Journal* **17**, 190–201.

Department of Health 1992: *Health of the Nation.* London: HMSO.

Department of Health 1994: *Health-promoting hospitals.* Leeds: NHS Management Executive.

Durrant, K. 1993: *The creative arts and the promotion of health in community settings.* Unpublished MSc Thesis, Leeds Metropolitan University, Leeds.

Faden, R.R. and Faden, A.I. 1978: The ethics of health education as public health policy. *Health Education Monographs* **6**, 180–97.

Freire, P. 1974: *Education and the practice of freedom.* London: Writers and Readers Publishing Co-operative (originally published in Portuguese in 1967).

Godfrey, C., Hardman, G. and Maynard, A. 1989: *Priorities for health promotion: an economic approach.* Discussion Paper 59. York: Centre for Health Economics, York University.

Goodman, R.M., Burdine, J.N., Meehan, E. and McLeroy, K.R. 1993: Special issue on community coalitions. *Health Education Research* **8**.

Green, L.W. and Lewis, F.M. 1986: *Measurement and evaluation in health education and health promotion.* Palo Alto, CA: Mayfield.

Hirst, P. 1969: The logic of the curriculum. *Journal of Curriculum Studies* **1**, 142–58.

Janz, N.K. and Becker, M.H. 1984: The health belief model: a decade later. *Health Education Quarterly* **11**, 1–47.

Jessor, R. and Jessor, S.L. 1977: *Problem behavior and psychosocial development: a longitudinal study of youth.* New York: Academic Press.

LeFanu, J. (ed.) 1994: *Preventionitis: the exaggerated claims of health promotion.* London: The Social Affairs Unit.

Ley, P. 1990: *Communicating with patients.* London: Chapman and Hall.

Lyng, S. 1990: Edgework: a social psychological analysis of voluntary risk taking. *American Journal of Sociology* **95**, 851–86.

Macleod Clark, J. 1993: From sick nursing to health nursing: evolution or revolution? In Wilson-Barnett, J. and Macleod Clark, J. (eds) *Research in health promotion and nursing.* London: Macmillan 256–70.

Macleod Clark, J., Kendall, S. and Haverty, S. 1990: Helping people to stop smoking: a study of the nurse's role. *Journal of Advanced Nursing* **15**, 357–63.

Mill, J.S. 1961: *On liberty* (reprinted in *Essential works of John Stuart Mill*). New York: Bantam Books.

Nutbeam, D. *et al.* 1991: *Youth health promotion: from theory to practice in school and community.* London: Forbes Publications.

Sarvela, P.D. and McDermott, R.J. 1993: *Health education evaluation and measurement: a practitioner's perspective.* Madison, WI: Brown & Benchmark.

Society of Public Health Educators 1976: *Code of Ethics, 15 October 1976.* San Francisco, CA: Society of Public Health Educators.

Tones, B.K. 1992: Health promotion, empowerment and the concept of control. In *Health education: politics and practice.* Victoria, Australia: Deakin University Press, 27–89.

Tones, B.K. 1993a: The importance of horizontal programmes in health education. *Health Education Research* **8**, 455–9.

Tones, B.K. 1993b: Changing theory and practice: trends in methods, strategies and settings in health education. *Health Education Journal* **52**, 126–39.

Tones, B.K. 1997: Health promotion: empowering choice. In Myers, L. and Midence, K. (eds), *Adherence to treatment.* Oxford: Oxford University Press, 783–814.

Tones, B.K. and Tilford, S. 1994: *Health education: effectiveness, efficiency and equity.* London: Chapman and Hall.

Tuckett, D. *et al.* 1985: *Meetings between experts.* London: Tavistock.

Vincent, M.L., Clearie, A.F. and Schluchter, M.D. 1987: Reducing adolescent pregnancy through school and community based education. *Journal of the American Medical Association* **257**, 3382–6.

Warner, K.E. 1989: Effects of the antismoking campaign: an update. *American Journal of Public Health* **79**, 144–51.

Whitehead, M. and Tones, B.K. 1990: *Avoiding the pitfalls.* London: Health Education Authority.

World Health Organization 1985: *Targets for Health for All.* Copenhagen: WHO Regional Office for Europe.

World Health Organization 1986: *Ottawa Charter for Health Promotion.* Copenhagen: WHO Regional Office for Europe.

World Health Organization 1991: *The Budapest Declaration on Health-Promoting Hospitals.* Business Meeting on Health Promoting Hospitals, 31 May–1 June 1991. Copenhagen: World Health Organization.

World Health Organization 1994: Adolescent girls face a dangerous crossroads in life, says WHO. Press Release WHO-70, 3 October 1994.

PART II

Empowerment of client groups

4

Empowering older people through communication

Andrée Le May

Setting the scene

This chapter focuses on the empowerment of older people through communication. Under this umbrella several key issues will be discussed, such as how communication can be enhanced for older people with challenged communication skills, how older people's voices can be heard in determining health care services or their quality, and how older people, through communication, may be able to guide research into issues which are central to maintaining their well-being. However, before considering these issues it is important to decide, first, if all older people need to be empowered, and then what empowerment and communication mean within the context of this chapter.

It seems sensible to assert that older people *per se* do not need empowering, as the majority are already empowered. Empowerment is a long-term process which occurs over time and does not simply begin in old age (Clark, 1989). The myth that older people are in some way disempowered has an ageist quality which is unacceptable and largely untrue. Most older people claim to be enjoying life, generally have good health, and do not experience extreme loneliness or dependency on others (Midwinter, 1991). However, a minority do experience problems in relation to these areas, and may consequently find that the empowering actions of health care practitioners can enhance their well-being. Some people belonging to these groups will value efforts to empower them through skilled communication, proposing alternative strategies for communication or encouraging them to voice their views; others will not. This chapter is written with this diversity in mind.

Both empowerment and communication have been ascribed various meanings during their rise to popular usage, and much debate surrounds their impact on a person's well-being. Frequently, authors and health care practitioners associate values with each of these terms, suggesting, for instance, that skilled communication may have a beneficial effect on an individual's physical, psychological and social well-being, and that empowerment may in turn be associated with a positive enabling outcome. In this chapter empowerment is viewed as 'enabling people to acquire the skills and self-confidence needed to bring about improvements in the quality of their lives, or helping people to compete more effectively for scarce resources' (Braye and Preston-Shoot, 1996, p. 50). Both of these definitions are relevant, since older people are a highly diverse section of the population with varying needs and differing perspectives on life.

Communication may be described as a complicated system in which a message passes from one person to another (or a group of people) through a series of differing verbal and non-verbal routes. Successful communication is a complex process which involves the transmission, recognition, comprehension and interpretation of verbal and non-verbal cues. Any alteration to a person's ability to undertake this process will result in compromised communication, which in turn may lead to feelings of reduced well-being and health. This is particularly relevant when older people are being considered, as they may, due to age- or illness-related challenges to communication, find their ability to communicate their views, feelings, needs or wishes to others changed. These changed abilities may be viewed as disempowering, and it is with this in mind that enhancing communication may be seen to be empowering.

Tones (1993, p. 5) suggests that the process of empowerment is one which is 'enabling and supporting rather than cajoling and coercing', and this can be coupled with the view that empowerment is 'essentially a process arising from valuing other people' (Chavasse, 1992, p. 2). It is natural, therefore, to suggest that empowerment is more likely to occur if there are shared understandings of the situation, and older people feel able to voice opinions with the certainty that these will be listened to and respected. Thus a clear link between empowerment and communication can be built which involves the establishment of a partnership between people.

Within the medical context, Clark (1996, p. 765) suggests that 'empowerment as partnership suggests that the principles of mutual understanding, dialogue and discussion necessary to create the shared meaning of an individual's life and health concerns lie at the core of a new clinical relationship between provider and patient.' These new relationships incorporate the features traditionally linked to empowerment, and may be facilitated through skilled communication. These include, as Roter and Hall (1992) propose, the sharing of the patient's story, treating patients as experts, valuing the patient's perspective and the practitioner's perspective, sharing information and expertise, reciprocity and understanding one another's changing role within the partnership.

The 1990s will be remembered for their many attempts to foster a culture which encourages partnerships at all levels between practitioners, purchasers of health care, patients and the general public (Farrell and Gilbert, 1996). This, together with many individual professions' efforts to alter the traditional balance of power within health care practitioner–patient relationships, and to promote sustainable partnerships, sets the backdrop for this chapter. Against this there is a clear commitment to communication between older people and their providers of health care, fuelled by the rapidly changing needs of older people, advancing health care techniques and changing health care environments (Clark, 1996) experienced during the last three decades. These issues have impacted on each other and contribute to the emergence of three relevant themes which are intuitively interlinked, namely empowerment, self-care and the right to self-determination and autonomy (Clark, 1996). These, again, serve to contextualize this chapter.

Taking nursing as an exemplar, partnerships may be developed which could result, for older people, in improved compliance, reduced dissatisfaction (Cook *et al.*, 1990), greater efficacy of health education, enhanced dignity and greater involvement in choosing appropriate approaches to health care or continuing care as a result of long-term frailty (Royal College of Nursing, 1996). However, it should be remembered that these partnerships will be tempered by certain factors, such as a person's knowledge, and his or her general health status or wish to become involved in the partnership (Biley, 1992; Hope, 1996), as well as specific individual traits which will influence the relationship between partners.

Factors which may influence partnerships

Factors such as age, gender, socio-cultural background and the context of the communication will all impact on communication and its potential for empowering older people. The literature suggests several differences, related to age in particular, which may influence the potential for empowering older people through communication when one partner is younger than another, as is often the case in health care settings. These may be referred to as intergenerational differences (Biggs, 1993), and they occur because older people have 'been socialized at a different time and to a different set of cultural imperatives' than those in the younger age groups (Dowd, 1986, p. 183). This cultural divide may result in things being associated with different values, meanings and consequences, as well as being done in different ways and for different reasons (Buchanan and Middleton, 1995). These differences may influence the process of communication in several ways.

- Young and old people have different roles to fulfil and are therefore likely to have differing values. This may be exacerbated by a tendency for people to prefer interacting with those whom they perceive in some way as equals, leading to reduced 'cross-age social interaction' (Dowd, 1986, p. 152), resulting in a lack of understanding of cross-generational experiences.

- Younger people may find it hard to understand older people's views and feelings, since they have not experienced either the life events associated with growing older, or the world in which the older person aged. Older people, whilst having the experience of being younger, experienced this in a different culture, thereby minimizing the potential for shared experiences; the world views of the young and old are consequently dissimilar even when they are living within the same time frame. This may make the establishment of an empowering partnership hard to achieve, since the mismatch of experiences may result in compromised opportunities for empathic communication and difficulty in understanding issues central to an older person's life (Clark, 1996).

- People from different generations, despite sharing the same 'language', may find that the meanings ascribed to certain words differ between generations, resulting in ambiguity. Conversations may also take on different structures and functions between generations, with older people placing more value on small talk, seeing it as a central component of relationship-building, whereas younger people may be more sceptical about the value of this element of communication (Giles and Coupland, 1991; Williams and Giles, 1996). Similarly, the more discursive style of older people may be seen by some as 'rambling', rather than as a skilled component of interesting conversation. These differences may lead to intolerance and again stunt the development of empowering partnerships. This may, although having the potential to influence all interactions, impact on the way in which health care practitioners and older people talk to each other (Roter and Hall, 1992) and therefore be of particular importance in the negotiation and maintenance of empowering partnerships.

- Nussbaum, *et al.* (1989) suggested that older people may be reluctant to communicate with younger people, particularly if this involves suggesting specific courses of action or seeking information. These findings have particular significance for empowerment, as the establishment of an equal partnership which promotes the sharing of information, in an attempt to facilitate choice, may be undermined.

- Health issues frequently dominate older people's conversations, emphasizing the importance of health (Giles and Coupland, 1991; Midwinter, 1991) and its association with old age, whereby feeling old may be directly associated with ill health (Williams, 1990). However, this may not always be the case, since many older people with chronic illness or disability still report that they 'feel good', suggesting a multifaceted view of health (Sidell, 1995). These views may not be shared or understood by younger people, and may therefore affect their ability to empathize with their older partners and vice versa.

- Old age can also be a time when illness- and age-related functional changes challenge communication specifically (e.g. impaired sight, hearing, speech or cognition) and therefore the maintenance of communication skills. This in turn may make it hard to sustain empowering partnerships with people of any age.

Further cultural issues which influence partnerships and empowerment through communication may be associated with status differences between partners, the nature and quality of any existing ties between partners, the reason for the partnership and the individual philosophy of each partner. These can be expressed in several ways and may profoundly affect interactions.

- Power differences related to professional status and age-related status may also occur and be worsened when practitioners stereotype older people as dependent, because they associate primarily with older people who require help (Biggs, 1993). These differences may also be affected by or affect the older person's attitude towards participating in medical decision-making and their relationships with health care practitioners (McWilliam *et al.*, 1994). Clark (1996, p. 748) suggests that communication, within the medical arena, 'represents a clash between two different "cultures" – one technical and scientific, the other embodying the lived reality of an older person.' Closing this gap is a central goal in empowering partnerships which acknowledge that in many instances the older person knows best about the impact of their health care problem on their values, wishes and goals (Clark, 1996). Both medicine, as Clark suggests, and nursing may find themselves trapped between 'the facts and values of practice, between the science and art of professionalism' (Clark, 1996, p. 750) when developing partnerships are considered. Establishing a shared meaning may be an important facet of empowerment through communication.
- The need for care may throw together people who would not usually interact, e.g. the nurse and the resident in a nursing home. This enforced 'partnership' may be made more difficult by the intimate nature of the care. Cook *et al.* (1990) suggested that communication is affected by the professional and personal characteristics of the health care practitioner, the patient and his or her family or friends. Continuing care is one area of care in which all of these people are involved in decision-making. This triad may complicate partnerships, as well as facilitating them, since conflicting opinions may be voiced. In these instances careful negotiation is required which continues to retain the focus of the interaction and enhance the development of empowering partnerships. Another more specific example of this tripartite partnership may be seen when the older person is suffering from dementia and is being cared for at home. In such a situation there is increasing evidence to suggest that the carer's needs should be addressed within the health care partnership to reduce

burnout (Almberg *et al.*, 1997) and provide support to both parties. Until recently, this represented good practice. However, current legislation emphasizes the need to consider carers more explicitly in decision-making than before (Department of Health, 1995), thus drawing them actively into the partnership.

- The underlying philosophy of any care facility is likely to have a marked impact on the quality of the partnerships created. Nussbaum *et al.* (1985) found that the individual nurse's philosophy of care also influenced his or her communication with older people living in nursing homes. They found that nurses who felt a high affinity towards residents were able to talk more about old times, religion and problems of old age, and to be more friendly and relaxed, thereby facilitating the formation of partnerships, than nurses who did not feel close to residents.

It is also likely that the type of presenting problem(s) faced by the older residents will guide this philosophy, e.g. if the older resident has an enduring mental health problem or dementia. A clear philosophy which empowers residents will be particularly appropriate under these circumstances, and will guide partnership-building through communication. One such approach has been adopted by The Retreat in York (Haywood and Scott, 1997), and may help to promote enhanced feelings of empowerment for the elderly residents with mental health problems. The philosophy states that residents have the right to:

> have the same human value as other members of society, irrespective of their degree of disability or dependence; have the same varied needs as other members of the community; have the same moral and legal rights as other citizens; have the right to forms of support which do not isolate them from family and friends; have a spiritual life that requires nurture and expression; are unique individuals with a distinctive pattern of capabilities and needs.
>
> (Haywood and Scott, 1997, p. 364)

This explicit philosophy, used in conjunction with that of the individual health care practitioner, may provide a useful framework for empowerment within individual partnerships.

All in all these differences and their consequences have the potential to influence empowerment markedly, through communication, when partners are of differing ages, health status and professional status and each needs serious consideration by all those involved in the provision of health care to older people.

Establishing partnerships

As the word partnership suggests, these relationships include an element of interdependency which will vary during the course of the partnership and is open to negotiation. The negotiation of partnerships between health care practitioners and patients may be described as the first step in the process of empowerment. Much has been written, in terms of policy statements, about this process during the 1990s, emphasizing the potential value of establishing partnerships as part of the movement towards consumerism within the health care sector (Farrell and Gilbert, 1996) and evidence-based patient choice (Hope, 1996). To take full advantage of these movements, all consumers, regardless of age, need to have sufficient information to make choices between alternatives, the ability to make these choices, the opportunity to exercise choice and the possibility of redress (Blaxter, 1993, cited by Farrell and Gilbert, 1996), coupled with the respect of their health care partners, thus encouraging informed choice (Farrell and Gilbert, 1996). These features are the key components of any partnership.

Focusing on nursing, Muetzel (1988, p. 98) describes partnership as a 'working association between two parties (who are not necessarily equals) in a joint enterprise, and which implies gains for both'. She suggests that partnerships between patients and nurses have always been present, but emphasizes that it is the balance of these relationships which is important. This observation still holds true. Christensen (1993) describes negotiating partnerships as a two-way process in which both the nurse and the patient have important contributions to make. For nurses these involve attending (being present, listening, ministering and comforting), enabling through coaching and encouraging, interpreting care and patient requirements, responding to situations as they occur, and anticipating what will happen to patients. The patients' work involves managing themselves and taking some responsibility for this, surviving the experience, affiliating with health care practitioners and interpreting the experience as it unfolds. Once the partnership has been negotiated, the work of the nurse and the patient centres on maintaining the partnership and steering a course through the experience which may involve each partner taking a lead at varying stages. For example, at the outset of a partnership the health care practitioner may take the lead in seeking out and providing relevant information, with the older person absorbing this knowledge. Later these roles may be reversed, particularly if the older person is suffering from a chronic problem, since, as time passes, he or she may become the expert in the partnership and provide new knowledge to the health care practitioner. This seemingly simplistic example shows the strength and far-reaching potential of empowerment through communication, since the growing partnership allows the older person to develop not only knowledge but also confidence to pass on new knowledge to the health care practitioner, suggesting a movement of power from one partner to the other. All of the stages in this partnership may be achieved through the use of sensitive communication skills.

The establishment of potentially empowering partnerships is important for all older people who require interventions to maintain or enhance their health status. The framework described by Christensen (1993) may generate short- or long-term partnerships and be particularly relevant in old age, when partnerships may extend over several years, as is the case for elderly people living in nursing or residential homes.

When longer term partnerships are considered, the qualities of the partnership become of paramount importance, since they are liable to influence the older partner's feelings of dignity, choice and individuality. In order to understand this better, Ford (1994), after interviewing older people, established several elements which older people felt to be central to the relationship between themselves and the nurses providing continuing care. These included sociability (civility, humour and socializing), reciprocity (friendship, sharing and solving problems) and the idea of 'being my nurse' (showing involvement, partnership, being a confidant and caring individually for each person), and they clearly show what some older people expect from partnerships with nurses.

Skilled communication, within empowering partnerships, has the potential to develop a rapport between the health care practitioner and the older person which builds trust, support and understanding as well as facilitating collaborative decision-making. Thus it provides older people with the opportunity to enhance their well-being and increase their level of participation in the health care process, as well as reinforcing the fact that older people are worthy of active involvement in partnerships. Thus in order to achieve empowering partnerships, we need to consider how we can:

- adjust the balance of the relationship between the professional and the patient or client;
- provide information to enable choice;
- respect choice;
- minimize manipulation; and
- maintain partnerships.

At the same time we must continually ask to what extent older people choose to become and remain involved in the process of empowerment. Empowerment is therefore intrinsically linked to the ability of a person to determine if and when he or she wishes to participate in an empowering partnership. All of these issues can be linked to communication, and therefore one may conjecture that communication is influential on the process of empowerment.

Empowering communication strategies

Although empowerment is not a simple strategy, but 'a fundamental way of thinking' (McDougall, 1997, p. 4), there are several communication strategies which may result in enhancing empowerment within a partnership which values unconditionally those involved in it. These are outlined below.

- *Acknowledge the older person's reality* in order to establish trust and respect. Nussbaum *et al.* (1989) warn against the use of statements which fail to acknowledge the older person's reality. These 'disconfirming' statements may make older people doubt themselves and their understanding of their own situation. This type of poor communication may stem from some of the intergenerational differences described earlier, and is likely to be disempowering. Examples of this include the use of patronizing, childish talk, or ignoring expressed viewpoints or feelings. It is important that health care practitioners are aware of the potentially deleterious effect of this kind of communication and understand that some older people associate disconfirmation with dementia and confusion, which in their turn are seen as disempowering and dehumanizing. Nussbaum *et al.* (1989) also suggest that older people may be disconfirming to the young, too, e.g. through forgetfulness. This is liable to affect partnerships, so it is essential that health care practitioners recognize this as potentially disempowering to both partners. Clark (1996) also suggests that within the clinical arena the reality of the patient's condition is, of necessity, redefined within the practitioner's discipline-based cognitive structures, thus having the potential to create a gap between the patient's reality and the practitioner's interpretation of it. This reshaped reality may lead to a disjointed representation of the patient's condition, needs and wishes with resultant inappropriate actions and diminished opportunities for partnership. To minimize these effects, Clark (1996, p. 752) advises practitioners of their 'responsibility to translate the patient's life-world statements into medical terms, and medical statements of problems into the patient's terms.' The ability to do this presents a challenge to all involved in the care of older people, and relies on the use of skilled, empowering communication strategies.
- *Avoid jargon and controlling language* (Hewison, 1995), since these will lessen equality within the partnership and may result in the older partner feeling ill-informed and frustrated, rather than empowered to make informed decisions. On the other hand, the oversimplification of language may make older people feel that they lack the ability to understand and so feel patronized; this again may have a detrimental effect on the partnership. Within encounters between older people and health care practitioners, language may influence the ability of either partner to establish the rapport which ensures that patients and practitioners are seen as equal partners.
- *Check out interpretations,* since young and old people may have different meanings for words, and misunderstandings will result in a reduction in trust within the partnership and limit opportunities for empowered decision-making. This may also occur as a result of conflicting world views, e.g. those of the physician and the older person. Matthews *et al.* (1993) emphasize the need to reduce stereotypic behaviours in order to

reach a shared understanding which combines the physician's science with the patient's reality. This process allows patients to be treated holistically with clear links being drawn between the presenting problem(s), the patient's world view and the health care practitioner's world view, thus preparing the ground for sustained partnerships.

- *Create an open atmosphere between interactors* which values the patient's beliefs and goals and avoids ritualistic or unrewarding conversations which are unlikely to increase knowledge or enhance well-being. Clark (1996) emphasizes the value of asking the older person to specifically discuss their needs, values and care preferences, thus making them feel that they are valued partners in the decision-making process.

- *Develop and use a variety of verbal and non-verbal communication skills.* In order to negotiate and sustain empowering partnerships it is essential that health care practitioners have well-developed skills in listening and watching their partners, since these will enable them to tune into the older person's needs effectively. These techniques may also help health care practitioners to identify and understand the range of their patients' needs. Wide-ranging questioning will help to establish rapport (Matthews *et al.*, 1993) and empathy, rather than using questions which focus narrowly on the presenting problem(s). Use the whole range of communication skills where appropriate (speech, eye contact, facial expression, gesture, body movement, touch, laughter, etc.) to create an understanding between partners. These may be augmented with specific techniques such as the inclusion of empathic statements, sharing experiences through self-disclosure, summarizing and re-presenting elements of conversations and using reinforcement.

- *Consider alternative forms of communication* (signing, using gestures, writing information down, pre-set movements to signify responses or the use of computerized communication systems), since many older people experience communication difficulties.

- *Provide appropriate sources of relevant information* which take into account any communication problems which may present themselves. Try to give information topic by topic rather than all at once, and make sure that you accurately assess the extent of the patient's knowledge prior to, and following, the giving of information. It is important to recognize that information may be presented formally and informally. Abley (1997) describes the former approach in her study of older people's use of inhalers following an education programme. In this study, 27 older people who were using inhalers in hospital enrolled in a teaching programme to improve their use of inhalers. Each person received four one-to-one teaching sessions from a nurse, and an information sheet on inhaler technique. Comparisons were made before and after the intervention to determine the effect of these formalized 'communications'. The results showed a significant improvement in technique following the programme, suggesting that interventions targeted towards enhancing technical ability, and therefore health status, are likely to empower older people by increasing their confidence and knowledge.

- *Check that communication aids work* and that the environment is conducive to communicating.
- *Consider using specific techniques*, for instance reminiscence (Holden, 1988), to lessen intergenerational barriers through shared conversations detailing backgrounds, experiences and attitudes. These may help to formulate a more appropriate understanding of the nature of ageing, the position of older people within society and the nature of care required, and indeed provided (Buchanan and Middleton, 1995), thus allowing health care professionals to understand and empathize with the variety of older people's experiences. On an individual basis, reminiscence may be useful in encouraging an older person to tell their story and thereby create the opportunity to reach appropriate shared decisions. On the other hand Buchanan and Middleton (1995) emphasize the need for caution since talking about the past may reinforce the cultural divide referred to earlier (Dowd, 1986). This technique may therefore be seen as a double-edged sword which may either reduce or increase inter-generational differences and consequently may have a profound effect on empowerment, which is dependent on the extent to which partners value each other (Chavasse, 1992).
- *Emphasize negotiation* by creating a partnership in which the older person and his or her carer(s) are able to negotiate approaches to care, leading to a mutually determined decision which can be implemented and evaluated. McCullough (1988) sets out a series of steps which may be used to create or improve communication. These include assessing the level of information already held by the older person and their understanding of it, correcting any deficits or misunderstandings, identifying the person's values, beliefs and goals in relation to care, negotiating the best way forward, and finally reaching a shared, mutually supported, realistic decision.

Enhancing older people's communication skills

The principal challenges to communication which are likely to impinge on this partnership are changes to visual, auditory, cognitive and vocal ability. Deficits in any of these will individually impact on empowerment in several different ways. However, if one challenge is accompanied by another, this will doubly disadvantage the older person and complicate the process of partnership.

In the case of visual impairment the effects may include limited orientation to the environment, compounded by the inability to distinguish non-verbal cues or focus on the written word, resulting in isolation and reduced opportunities for interaction between partners or with others outside the partnership. Similarly far-reaching effects may result from auditory incapacity, since hearing impairment may result in the misinterpretation of messages, which may lead to embarrassment, fear, inappropriate responses and self-imposed isolation. Since many older people experience age-related changes in visual and auditory acuity, each of these may influence partnerships and result in limited opportunities for empowerment when the whole gamut of communication is considered. The net result has the potential to impact markedly on one-to-one interactions, group interactions and the ability to gather information to make choices or provide information regarding the quality of the partnership or the service provided.

Cognitive changes present complex communication problems which may lead to poor comprehension, limited vocabulary, inappropriate use of words, wandering from the subject or becoming mute. Written skills may also be compromised, limiting further opportunities for communication, and difficulties associated with comprehension may reduce the older person's capacity to understand information, thus reducing the scope for empowerment. Several language difficulties present in older age, and each of these will affect the older person's feelings of empowerment and the partnership within which empowerment is encouraged. Language disorders are likely to alter a person's ability to speak coherently, his or her self-confidence and his or her ability to assimilate or provide information. Profound cognitive and language changes are usually illness related, and this dimension will add an extra complexity to the partnership. Alterations in both of these abilities, whether presented singly or in conjunction with each other, will present major challenges for both partners which may minimize the realistic possibility of empowering older people through verbal communication.

Whilst acknowledging the profound impact of these altered abilities on the partnership and the effects of communication from all partners' perspectives, there are some useful general steps which may be taken to minimize the detrimental effects of these challenges and to maximize the potential for empowering communication between partners. These include:

- assessing the extent of the deficit and how this affects both partners;
- checking that communication aids (e.g. spectacles, hearing aids) are available, in working order and used;
- monitoring the effectiveness of communication aids;
- considering whether referral for assessment is necessary;
- creating an environment that is conducive to communication;
- using clear, accessible language augmented with relevant non-verbal communication;
- considering alternative communication strategies (e.g. sign language, drawing, picture boards);
- encouraging involvement in order to minimize isolation.

More specific approaches which address each of the challenges outlined above are detailed in Gravell (1988) and Le May (1998), whilst an up-to-date, systematic review of the literature related to the role of communication in nursing care for elderly people has been undertaken by Caris-Verhallen *et al.* (1997), which may prove useful to all health care practitioners.

Hearing older people's voices – a necessary component of health care provision

Partnerships may also be seen more globally, suggesting a relationship between providers of health and social care and the public. In these instances the partnership takes on a different quality, although the emphasis remains on the exchange of information in order to make informed choices. Hope (1996) identifies numerous mechanisms for facilitating this, including the media, general education, health shops, patient groups, health care professionals, videos, interactive videos, the Internet and books/booklets from libraries and bookshops. Clearly, not all older people will have access to this range of resources, but the breadth of information available will help each person to feel more powerful in making choices, and will increase the likelihood of empowerment, at a more collective level, through the communication of information.

Despite the increased availability of information, older people are often viewed as a silent majority due to their reluctance to voice their needs for and opinions of health care. Various explanations have been put forward to explain this, ranging from the assumption held by both older people and some health care practitioners that old age inevitably brings poor health (Fennell *et al.*, 1991) to a lack of understanding of older people's needs due to a lack of knowledge, from research and experience, of their health needs and service requirements. These are likely to remain important since the number of older people is increasing together with an increased complexity of health and illness associated with older age. If we are to provide comprehensive care which meets older people's needs, their opinions should be actively canvassed and their voices heard.

Health care practitioners may facilitate this by providing older people with opportunities to voice their views individually or collectively through various fora (Copperman and Morrison, 1995), or by involving them in working groups to plan specific care initiatives or research priorities. Several specific approaches have been suggested as means for canvassing the views of older consumers of health care. Collective approaches include access to Health Authorities, Trusts, Community Health Councils, pensioners' groups, support groups and organizations specifically concerned with issues related to older age. More individual approaches may involve the use of data collected routinely through existing services but reconfigured for a different purpose. One potential area for expansion in this way is the 75-plus assessment undertaken through the General Practitioner services. This assessment has considerable scope for developing long-term partnerships which empower older people to review and maintain their health, use the services available and determine unmet individual needs. This information, collected on an individual basis, could be reconfigured on a practice-by-practice basis to review the collective needs and opinions of older clients, thereby ensuring that older people's voices are heard and are influential in the strategic management of the service. The development of this type of empowering partnership is likely to increase the provision of appropriate, equitable, cost-effective health care for older people, whilst continuing to acknowledge their diversity, in contrast to the present patchwork of services put together by various isolated disciplines (Royal College of Physicians, 1994).

Whilst the provision of services for older people is high on the health care agenda, the goal of empowering older people through communication is multifaceted, and should be approached in a variety of different ways, each supporting the others. In order to achieve this, service providers may need explicit strategies to strengthen their determination to canvass older people's views. One such approach, designed to empower older people to speak out, has been proposed by the Health Education Authority (Nelson, 1997). It recommends:

- the creation and maintenance of partnerships with other agencies to develop a national policy for promoting the health of older people;
- co-ordination of research and development on promoting health;
- promoting older people's involvement in the development of policies and services which create opportunities for partnership.

Care providers may find this a useful adjunct to the general move towards consumer involvement expressed through central policy during the 1990s.

Although the increased emphasis on consumerism has been complemented by equal attention to health promotion in later life, there remain some bizarre examples where age-related policies compromise empowerment. This is illustrated by the example of screening older women for breast cancer. Age Concern (1996) suggested that the present system failed to reach those women most at risk of breast cancer, namely those aged 65 years and over, since routine invitations for screening are not issued to this group. One may wonder why this occurs, and the sceptics among us may immediately consider a link between health promotion, disease detection and resource management. However, there are other persuasive answers which should not be discounted and which focus on the trajectory of the disease, since breast cancer is 'assumed' to be less aggressive in older age, and older women are more likely to die of other causes before malignancy itself causes death (Fentiman, 1994). Whilst these reasons are seductive, we need, if we are concerned with providing choice for older women, to consider canvassing their opinions at an individual and/or collective level, in order to facilitate more client-centred services for both providers and recipients of care. Age Concern (1996) commissioned a national survey of 1033 older women to assess their knowledge of screening programmes and the risks of breast cancer. The findings showed that few women thought themselves to be at high risk of developing breast cancer (24 per cent) or knew about their right to ask for screening. Simultaneously a survey was conducted in Hampshire (Age Concern, 1996) drawing on the views of 350 women. Of this group, 61 per cent did not know that they could request screening (40 per cent of whom planned to be screened in the future), and only 54 per cent regularly practised breast self-examination. These findings suggest that there is considerable scope not only to canvass older women's views, but also to provide more information to enable them to make informed choices regarding this element of health care.

If older people are to feel empowered, they need to feel able to be involved in all stages of the decision-making process, from policy decisions to individual decisions. However, in some instances health care providers (individually or collectively) may be less well placed to encourage commentary from older people than from other lay volunteer helpers. Dunning (1995) describes the value of the citizen advocate for older people who may be unable to represent their own interests or views. He defines citizen advocacy as

> a one-to-one ongoing partnership between a trained volunteer citizen advocate and a person who is not in a strong position to exercise or defend his or her rights and is at risk of being mistreated or excluded. The citizen advocate should be free from conflicts of interest with those providing services to their partner and should represent the interests of their partner as if they were their own.
>
> (Dunning, 1995, p. 20)

This approach will complement the concepts of partnership between individual health care practitioners and older people as well as those created at the more collective provider/purchaser level of care. Dunning suggests that citizen advocacy with older people has grown for several reasons, including recent changes in the approach to community care and increased reliance on institutional care within residential or nursing homes. Whilst these have provided greater opportunities for consumer involvement, there has been an increased reliance on members of the family, many of whom are themselves elderly, to provide care in the community, which has the potential to lead to feelings of exploitation and exhaustion. These potential accompaniments of old age are set against an increased amount of bureaucracy associated with health and social care, and a burgeoning of information regarding services, treatment options and the rights of the consumer, all of which need careful negotiation which could be facilitated through skilled empowering communication.

There still remain some groups of older people whose views are underrepresented. One example of this is the under-representation of the views of older people from ethnic minority groups, which may result in feelings of disempowerment at both an individual and a collective level. Whilst specific surveys have been undertaken to seek the views of black and ethnic minority groups (e.g. Health Education Authority, 1995), and their elders (Askham, 1995) increased attention needs to be paid to empowering these older people to speak out about their health care needs, the service provision which they experience and their level of satisfaction with it. Another example with the potential for under-representation of views may be those older people living within continuing care facilities. Increasingly, the favoured option for empowering communication in these settings has become the patients' or residents' committee (Millard and Kist, 1997; Sander, 1997), which has arisen from a philosophy which emphasizes that 'residents should run their own lives as far as possible' (Sander, 1997, p. 341).

Providers of health and social care have a responsibility to determine local needs and to publish their plans to meet these needs. If older people's views were to be systematically canvassed and included in these strategic plans, this would provide a potential mechanism for communication between consumer and provider which reflects the older person's perspective and supports the notion of partnership between service providers and consumers. However, in relation to this Braye and Preston-Shoot (1996, p. 119) emphasize that 'Services must be negotiated within the context of overt recognition of the power relationship between user and service provider, in a partnership that is more than just token recognition of a user's preference and within which every attempt has been made to empower the user's perspective.' The uncertainty with which providers of health care view consultation and consumerism should not be underestimated, and is exposed by the suggestion of Lupton *et al.* (1995) that empowered communication may threaten service providers' (and purchasers') power. This will result in a need to pay increased attention to facilitating older consumers' involvement, since 'the window of opportunity for public involvement in the NHS appears to be barely open' (Lupton *et al.*, 1995, p. 225) and some traditional mechanisms for voicing opinion, e.g. the Community Health Council, are threatened by changed priorities and roles (Lupton *et al.*, 1995).

Quality assurance – a mechanism for communicating older people's opinions of care

Since purchasers and providers of health care are continuously urged to consider service users' viewpoints and to evaluate the quality of their service, it is worth considering how the two can be merged to canvass older consumers' opinions. However, in order for this to be achieved realistically, all aspects of care assessment should involve consumer evaluations, as evidenced by Farrell and Gilbert's (1996, p. 9) suggestion that 'If quality policies are to be serious tools for effecting patient empowerment, they will have to pay much greater attention to the patient's view of clinical aspects of care'. However, this view may be met with scepticism, since audit takes a traditionally positivistic stance in which only measurable factors are worth considering, thus leading to the exclusion of patients' experiences and a devaluing of their input to service provision and development (Farrell and Gilbert, 1996).

One way of facilitating both the evaluation of services and the involvement of older people may be through the use of a variety of approaches to quality determination, ranging from retrospective patient satisfaction surveys to patient involvement in the concurrent evaluations of their care experiences. This variety of approach may thus increase the value of the patient experience in relation to the outcome of care. These techniques could therefore be used to initiate changes in the quality of the service to meet older people's needs, as well as empowering older people to communicate their opinions. This latter point is critical to establishing informed partnerships with older service users, since we cannot assume that service providers 'know best' through their observations and experiences of care.

The challenge to health care practitioners and planners is to consider ways of facilitating this level of empowering communication. Norman (1997), in his review of approaches to assessing quality in the care of older people, highlights several appropriate techniques. These range from methods which involve the older person in care evaluations (e.g. QUALPACS and Senior Monitor) to a six-stage clinical audit cycle (Smith, 1989) which explicitly involves the recipients of care and therefore has the hallmarks of establishing evaluative partnerships. These approaches facilitate the canvassing of older people's experiences of the services provided, whether as consumer or as carer of a consumer, and may also strengthen older people's feelings of control.

Health care practitioners and planners cannot work in isolation or assume that they can voice older people's views or experiences themselves, as is shown by the following quotation from a nurse working on a rehabilitation unit for older people:

> We thought we understood how patients felt, we thought we knew the problems they were experiencing, but every day the patients came up with things we had not thought about. It is a very humbling experience.
> (Copperman and Morrison, 1995, p. 41)

It is therefore vitally important to involve older consumers in the assessment of the quality of their care, since they are the only ones with the knowledge and experience to point out areas with which they are satisfied or those that require improvement.

Research – a mechanism for communicating older people's priorities

There is a growing recognition that consumer involvement in determining research priorities makes a valuable contribution to health and social care (Farrell and Gilbert, 1996). This is fuelled by the continued emphasis on evidence-based care and policy determination which provides the potential to canvass openly older people's views on research priorities and their inclusion in research projects. Canvassing the views of older people in relation to the selection of research priorities will ensure that research studies and their findings are perceived as relevant and do not ignore consumers' needs. This may be further enhanced by involving older people as lay members of Ethics Committees, which will contribute to establishing an understanding of what older people themselves perceive as important ethical issues in the conduct and utilization of research. These views, together with the results of empirical studies, may be used to influence the construction of a health and social care research agenda reflective of the diversity of older people's needs.

However, these ideals are set against a background which has acknowledged several barriers to the study of ageing populations. These range from the difficulties in undertaking certain types of research designs (e.g. longitudinal studies may be difficult to complete because of the potential shortage of study time, whilst difficulties may be experienced recruiting older people to experimental studies due to the multiple pathologies and polypharmacy often associated with illness in old age) to the consideration of ethical issues in relation to physical and mental frailty and informed consent (Butler, 1990). Viewed together, these issues severely restrict the amount and type of research in which older people may participate. This may in turn restrict the knowledge base for the provision of the complex care often necessitated at this stage of a person's life.

Research studies which address the complicated issues of ageing and the effects of disease will enhance knowledge and our ability to empathize with older people. The findings from this type of study are likely to influence the negotiation and maintenance of partnerships, and to shed light on ways of empowering older people through communication. An example of one such study is presented by Parr *et al.* (1997) through their investigation of 50 aphasic patients' experiences of stroke and its long-term consequences. The findings of this novel study are reported from the perspective of the aphasic subject, and emphasize the complexity of interactions between health care practitioners and clients. They highlight the need to build empowering partnerships to enable people with aphasia to cope with the far-reaching consequences of this long-term outcome of acute illness. Involvement in research – through commissioning, scrutinizing or participation – may actively empower older people to communicate their experiences, identify their research priorities and contribute to the enhancement of quality of life in older age.

Conclusions

Empowerment is a long-term process which, within health and social care settings, is often associated with complex service as well as relational issues. Empowering older people through skilled communication may enhance their feelings of control and involvement in individual treatment/care decisions, planning service provision, evaluating services and determining research priorities. Empowerment is dependent on the degree and quality of the communication at an individual and/or collective level, and the complexity of this process should not be underestimated but taken forward as a challenge worthy of attention by all service users and providers. This area is ripe for research in the future in order to determine the extent to which older people find skilled communication empowering, the factors which facilitate or hinder this, and the extent to which this diverse group of voices is heard when the health care agenda is set.

References

Abley, C. 1997: Teaching elderly patients how to use inhalers. A study to evaluate an education programme on inhaler technique, for elderly patients. *Journal of Advanced Nursing* **25**, 699–708.

Age Concern 1996: *Not at my age: why the present breast screening system is failing women aged 65 or over.* London: Age Concern.

Almberg, B., Grafstrom, M. and Winblad, B. 1997: Caring for a demented elderly person – burden and burnout among caregiving relatives. *Journal of Advanced Nursing* **25**, 109–16.

Askham, J. 1995: *Social and health authority services for elderly people from black and minority ethnic communities.* London: HMSO.

Biggs, S. 1993: *Understanding ageing.* Buckingham: Open University Press.

Biley, F. 1992: Some determinants that affect patient participation in decision-making about nursing care. *Journal of Advanced Nursing* **17**, 414–21.

Blaxter, M. 1993: *Consumer issues within the NHS.* NHS Research and Development Workshop. Unpublished discussion paper.

Braye, S. and Preston-Shoot, M. 1996: *Empowering practice in social care.* Buckingham: Open University Press.

Buchanan, K. and Middleton, D. 1995: Voices of experience: talk, identity and membership in reminiscence groups. *Ageing and Society* **15**, 457–91.

Butler, A. 1990: Research ethics and older people. In Peace, S. (ed.), *Researching social gerontology.* London: Sage, 162–70.

Caris-Verhallen, W., Kerkstra, A. and Bensing, J. 1997: The role of communication in nursing care for elderly people: a review of the literature. *Journal of Advanced Nursing* **25**, 915–33.

Chavasse, J. 1992: New dimensions of empowerment in nursing – and challenges. Guest editorial. *Journal of Advanced Nursing* **17**, 1–2.

Christensen, J. 1993: *Nursing partnership. A model for nursing practice*. Edinburgh: Churchill Livingstone.

Clark, P. 1989: The philosophical foundation of empowerment: implications for geriatric health care programs and practice. *Journal of Aging and Health* **1**, 2667–85.

Clark, P. 1996: Communication between provider and patient: values, biography, and empowerment in clinical practice. *Ageing and Society* **16**, 747–74.

Cook, M., Coe, R. and Hanson, K. 1990: Physician–elderly patient communication: processes and outcomes of medical encounters. In Stahl, S. (ed.), *The legacy of longevity*. Newbury Park: Sage, 291–309.

Copperman, J. and Morrison, P. 1995. *We thought we knew ... involving patients in nursing practice*. London: King's Fund Centre.

Department of Health 1995: *Carers (Recognition and Service) Act 1995*. London: HMSO.

Dowd, J. 1986: The old person as stranger. In Marshall, V. (ed.), *Later life. The social psychology of aging*. Beverly Hills, CA: Sage.

Dunning, A. 1995: *Citizen advocacy with older people: a code of good practice*. London: Centre for Policy on Ageing.

Farrell, C. and Gilbert, H. 1996: *Health care partnerships*. London: King's Fund.

Fennell, G., Phillipson, C. and Evers, H. 1991: *The sociology of old age*. Buckingham: Open University Press.

Fentiman, I. 1994: *Health Select Committee, 1994, Breast Cancer Services*. London: HMSO.

Ford, P. 1994: *What older people, as patients in continuing care, value in nurses*. Unpublished MSc Thesis, Keele University, Keele.

Giles, H. and Coupland, N. 1991: *Language: contexts and consequences*. Milton Keynes: Open University Press.

Gravell, R. 1988: *Communication problems in elderly people: practical approaches to management*. Beckenham: Croom Helm.

Haywood, S. and Scott, B. 1997: The Retreat experience: continuity and change in the care of older mentally ill people. In Denham, M. (ed.), *Continuing care for older people*. Cheltenham: Stanley Thornes, 360–71.

Health Education Authority 1995: *Toward better health service provision for black and minority ethnic groups*. London: Health Education Authority.

Hewison, A. 1995: Nurses' power in interactions with patients. *Journal of Advanced Nursing* **21**, 75–82.

Holden, U. 1988: Recognising the problems. In Holden, U. (ed.), *Neuropsychology and ageing*. London, Croom Helm, 1–22.

Hope, T. 1996: *Evidence-based patient choice*. London: King's Fund.

Le May, A. 1998: Communication skills. In Redfern, S. and Ross, F. (eds.), *Nursing elderly people*. Edinburgh: Harcourt Brace (in press).

Lupton, C., Buckland, S. and Moon, G. 1995: Consumer involvement in health care purchasing: the role and influence on community health care councils. *Health and Social Care in the Community* **3**, 215–26.

McCullough, L. 1988: An ethical model for improving the patient–physician relationship. *Inquiry* **25**, 454–68.

McDougall, T. 1997: Patient empowerment: fact or fiction? *Mental Health Nursing* **17**, 4–5.

McWilliam, C., Brown, J., Carmichael, J. and Lehman, J. 1994: A new perspective on threatened autonomy in elderly persons: the disempowering process. *Social Science and Medicine* **38**, 327–38.

Matthews, D., Suchman, A. and Branch, W. 1993: Making 'connexions': enhancing the therapeutic potential of the patient–clinician relationship. *Annals of Internal Medicine* **118**, 973–7.

Midwinter, E. 1991: *The British Gas report on attitudes to ageing.* London: British Gas.

Millard, P. and Kist, P. 1997: The Bolingbroke Hospital long-term care project. In Denham, M. (ed.), *Continuing care for older people.* Cheltenham: Stanley Thornes, 323–37.

Muetzel, P. 1988: Therapeutic nursing. In Pearson, A. (ed.), *Primary nursing: nursing in the Burford and Oxford Nursing Development Units.* London: Croom Helm, 89–116.

Nelson, F. 1997: Adopting a more mature approach. *Healthlines* **April**, 14–16.

Norman, I. 1997: Assessing quality in the care of older people: a review of approaches. *Health Care in Later Life* **2**, 26–45.

Nussbaum, J., Robinson, J. and Grew, D. 1985: Communicative behavior of the long-term health care employee: implications for the elderly resident. *Communication Research Reports* **2**, 16–22.

Nussbaum, J., Thompson, T. and Robinson, J. 1989: *Communication and aging.* New York: Harper & Row.

Parr, S., Byng, S. and Gilpin, S. 1997: *Talking about aphasia.* Buckingham: Open University Press.

Roter, D. and Hall, J. 1992: *Doctors talking with patients: patients talking with doctors.* Westport: Auburn House.

Royal College of Nursing 1996: *Nursing homes: nursing values.* London: Royal College of Nursing.

Royal College of Physicians 1994: *Ensuring equity of care for older people.* London: Royal College of Physicians.

Sander, R. 1997: Jubilee House. In Denham, M. (ed.), *Continuing care for older people.* Cheltenham: Stanley Thornes, 338–47.

Sidell, M. 1995: *Health in old age: myth, mystery and management.* Buckingham: Open University Press.

Smith, H. 1989: *Commitment to quality: safeguarding quality of care in long-stay psychiatric hospitals.* Discussion Paper 89/44. London: King's Fund.

Tones, K. 1993: The theory of health promotion: implications for nursing. In Wilson-Barnett, J. and Macleod Clark, J. (eds), *Research in health promotion and nursing.* Basingstoke: Macmillan, 3–12.

Williams, A. and Giles, H. 1996: Intergenerational conversations: young adults' retrospective accounts. *Human Communication Research* **2**, 220–50.

Williams, R. 1990: *The Protestant legacy: attitudes to death and illness among older Aberdonians.* Oxford: Oxford University Press.

5

Women sex workers, health promotion and HIV

Graham Scambler and Annette Scambler

Introduction

The degree of interest generated over the centuries by the institution of prostitution or, to use the designation we prefer, the 'sex industry', is perhaps unsurprising. Equally predictable has been the focus, largely if not exclusively by male scholars, commentators and enthusiasts, on female sex workers. Despite an unbroken historical presence, male sex workers have remained inconspicuous almost to the point of invisibility, to the extent that use of the terms 'prostitute' or 'sex worker' is automatically associated with women. This pattern has been essentially reproduced in the moral panic and AIDS-related research programmes of the 1980s and 1990s, although some systematic attention is now also being paid to male sex workers (see Davies and Feldman, 1997).

It is the brief of this contribution to review and reflect upon our own and others' work on women rather than men sex workers in what has sometimes been termed the 'AIDS era' (Scambler et al., 1990). In the opening section we make a number of points about the size and properties of the population of women sex workers in the UK, stressing heterogeneity and the various hazards associated with stereotyping. In the second section we review the literature, much of it epidemiological, on HIV infection and AIDs among women sex workers, and look also at the evidence relating to other sexually transmitted diseases (STDs), to drugs, to violence and abuse, and to more general and mundane threats to the health and well-being of women in the sex industry. The third section contains an account and critique of existing health care facilities for women sex workers, extending beyond primary and secondary services to outreach and health promotion. The fourth section explicates the concept of empowerment and underlines its susceptibility to use as a rhetorical device in political argument. In the final summing up, attention is concentrated on the potential for alternative future strategies to enhance effectively the health and proper care of women sex workers.

A social profile of women sex workers

What is striking about those who enter the sex industry, either as casual workers or as career workers, is their heterogeneity. To appreciate workers' diversity of backgrounds, motivations, experiences and aspirations is to resist conventional stereotypes of the sex worker (O'Neill, 1997; Scambler, 1997). These stereotypes home in on the conspicuous street worker: 'We are portrayed as women who stand on street corners, who wear microscopic miniskirts, who are foul-mouthed junkies, who are violent, with severe psychiatric disorders, and who were abused as kids' (Barbara, 1993). In fact, as Boyle (1994) emphasizes, street workers constitute the visible tip of an iceberg, with perhaps as much as nine-tenths of the sex trade – indoor workers – being 'hidden'. Nor can street workers be so easily and summarily characterized.

Stereotypical notions surrounding the 'whore stigma' have been analysed in detail elsewhere (Pheterson, 1993). All that is needed here is to rehearse selected 'theses' which together counter most of the worst excesses of this stigma and of the stereotyping of sex workers. Before doing this, however, it might be helpful to note briefly what has been called the 'paradox of attention' (Scambler, 1997). This maintains that much of the notoriety and interest generated with regard to the sex industry is a function less of what sex workers do than of the attention paid to it and of the projects of those who are paying it attention. Many of the familiar objections to sex work, for example, feminist and non-feminist arguments alike, apply equally well to other forms of work to which far less attention and indignation are directed. In reality, women sex workers and the lives they lead are far more mundane than is implied in the excesses of attention and stereotype. They are for the most part ordinary women who are systematically and ideologically misrepresented – in line with the projects of those who do so – as extraordinary.

The first thesis offered here reiterates the importance of heterogeneity. It is not just that only a minority of sex workers ply their trade openly on the streets. Contrary to the popular stereotype as well, most sex workers are not vulgar or immoral, nor do most of them live or work in social milieux plagued by habitual drug use, violence, anomie and hopelessness. As one university-educated escort worker explained to us, most women in the industry are invisible off-street workers, many of them autonomous and canny enough to evade public labelling (and even self-labelling) as social misfits and outsiders. In defiance of the homogeneity projected by public stereotype and mythology, women sex workers are, like most other groups of workers, mixed.

The second thesis is that it is both a caricature and erroneous to assume that sex workers are passive 'victims' of their socio- or psychopathological circumstances. This presumption of what Naffine (1987) terms 'gender-prescribed passivity' is quite unjustified. There is no reason to believe that sex workers are any less active and independent than any other group of female workers. They may in fact exercise a greater degree of control during their encounters with clients than many other female workers. This is of course of direct relevance to their potential as health educators (see below). There is evidence, too, that they typically experience more control over clients than rent-boys (Perkins and Bennett, 1985). Women sex workers should thus be seen as active, autonomous agents unless and until there is evidence to the contrary.

The third thesis debunks the myth that sex workers lack moral sensibility or commitment. One off-street worker made the point to us that 'we have our ethical code, just like doctors; it's no different'. It is clear from multiple ethnographic accounts that women commonly develop their own codes of practice to govern a range of practical behaviours from condom use to acceptable and unacceptable sexual requests. No longer is it appropriate to assume that sex workers are any more inclined to infringe against social norms or laws – with the exception of those specifically designed to limit their capacity to provide professional, rather than amateur, sexual services – than other people.

Fourthly, sex workers' reflexivity needs to be stressed. It is important to recognize not only the inadequacy of stereotyping them as passive victims of their backgrounds, but also the skill, expertise, resourcefulness and insight required to carry out their jobs profitably and safely. Most women quickly learn about the demands and hazards of sex work, and no less rapidly have any preconceptions they might have had prior to entering the sex industry of the hypocrisy and fallibility of 'respectable' men reinforced. Many are able to offer succinct and graphic accounts of core personifications and mechanisms of patriarchy out of work experience.

The fifth and final thesis draws attention to an innovative aspect of women sex workers' norm-breaking. Giddens (1992) argues that a new potential to challenge patriarchal structures and systems of beliefs and values has arisen through a combination of factors, one of the most important of which is 'plastic sexuality'. This refers to sexuality freed from its intrinsic relationship to production. Plastic sexuality, Giddens contends, was a precondition of the sexual revolution of recent years. The principal gains have been in female sexual autonomy and in the flourishing of gay culture. These gains constitute a considerable challenge to what Brittan (1989) calls 'hierarchic heterosexuality'.

It has been argued that women sex workers have contributed to sexual emancipation. The longstanding sex worker activist Helen Buckingham explained to Silver that:

I challenged the current supposition that men could have women when they felt like it, with no obligation, and that women enjoyed the sex, enjoyed giving themselves, enjoyed being walked over, enjoyed being used, enjoyed being disposed of. They thought that this is all part of the feminine personality: women are masochistic by nature and they like this. And to meet a woman who said, 'No, I'm not like that and I don't like it, but this is a bloody good way to earn a living' was terribly, terribly threatening.

(Silver, 1993, p. 78)

A bolder claim might be that women sex workers manage to integrate plastic sexuality with the reflexive project of self. It is autonomy and reciprocity that are pivotal here. It is certainly true that some women *choose* the rewards that attend sex work, like higher pay than most women and many men in more orthodox employment, foreign travel, and unusual freedom over working hours – and some clearly enjoy (aspects of) their work (French, 1988). It should be noted, too, that although the sex industry remains deeply symptomatic of patriarchy, this does not prevent most women sex workers from controlling most of their encounters with most of their clients. In so far as this is the case, there is resistance to patriarchy even here.

These theses add up to the contention that any examination of the sex industry should start from the *assumption* that women are individualistic, active and wilful, moral, reflexive and insightful, as well as potential innovators with respect to patriarchal norms. This necessarily involves confronting the paradox of attention. What cannot be denied, however, is that some women, even if only a small minority, conform precisely to the popular stereotype of the sex worker. Nor should it be forgotten that sex work can be dangerous, leave profound emotional scars and, in exceptional circumstances, lead to loss of life (Scambler, 1997).

Sex work, HIV and health status

Much of the recent and more systematic research on the health status of women sex workers has been either prompted by, or a side-effect of, media-generated moral panic surrounding AIDs, dating from the mid-1980s. Its focus has tended to be epidemiological, and its brief to chart the prevalence of HIV infection. The picture that has emerged is less alarming than many moral entrepreneurs predicted.

A multicentre cross-sectional survey of women sex workers across nine European societies reported an overall prevalence of 1.5 per cent in non-intravenous drug users (non-IVDU) and 31.8 per cent in intravenous drug users (IVDU) (European Working Group on HIV Infection in Female Prostitutes, 1993). A total of 79 London women were tested as part of this survey, three of whom were IVDU, and none tested positive. In a larger London series, Ward, Day and their colleagues reported overall prevalence rates for HIV of 1.7 per cent for 1986–1988, and 0.9 per cent for 1989–1991 (Barton *et al.*, 1987; Day *et al.*, 1988; Ward *et al.*, 1993). Infection in these women was related either to injecting drug use or to sex with a non-paying partner known to have HIV.

Not all estimates of HIV prevalence are as low as these figures for London, and there is in fact considerable variation. While in Sheffield, in 1986–1987, no women sex workers were found to be HIV-seropositive (Woolley *et al.*, 1988), in Glasgow in 1991 it was found that 2.5 per cent were infected with HIV (McKeganey *et al.*, 1992), and in Edinburgh in 1988, 14 per cent were reported to be infected with HIV (Morgan Thomas *et al.*, 1990). The higher prevalence in Edinburgh reflects both the inclusion of male sex workers in the sample and the high local rate of IVDU. Numerous studies conducted in the UK, Europe and North America have confirmed that women sex workers with a history of IVDU are at highest risk of HIV.

If women sex workers who are IVDU and share equipment experience an enhanced risk of HIV, those who are non-IVDU may also be at increased risk through their sexual contacts, either with clients or with non-paying partners. This risk is, of course, reduced by consistent condom use or by the avoidance of penetrative sex. Ward *et al.* (1993) found that the proportion of women who reported always using condoms for vaginal sex with clients rose from just under 50 per cent in 1985 to 98 per cent in 1990. However, the rate of condom use tends to be lower with regular than with casual clients, and lower still with non-paying partners. Given that some partners may be IVDU and/or be having unprotected sex with other women, it may be – paradoxically in view of the moral panic fuelled by the media – that while clients generally remain protected through consistent condom use, women sex workers are themselves at risk of HIV infection from their partners. Moreover, since the presence of condoms is as important as a symbolic barrier between women and their clients as their absence is important for worthwhile intimacy with non-paying partners, this problem admits of no easy solution (Day *et al.*, 1987). Interestingly, the same pattern has been found with male sex workers (Davies and Feldman, 1997).

Ward and Day summarize HIV risk as follows:

> women working as prostitutes report high levels of condom use in commercial sex, but remain at some risk of HIV from injecting drug use and from unprotected sex with non-paying partners. At present these two factors have not led to high levels of HIV infection.
>
> (Ward and Day, 1997, p. 142)

However, the same authors provide evidence of rather higher rates of other sexually transmitted infections. For example, 44 per cent of women interviewed in 1989–1991 reported a past history of gonorrhoea (Ward *et al.*, 1993). In Sheffield, Woolley *et al.* (1988) found that 28 per cent of women had at least one episode of gonorrhoea during 1986–1987, and 24 per cent had chlamydia.

Other health problems considered to characterize women sex workers include drug use and injury or abuse. The rate of use of tobacco, alcohol and illicit drugs such as cannabis by women sex workers can be high. In a study in Edinburgh, for example, it was found that 87 per cent of women sex workers smoked. Of those who had drunk alcohol in the week prior to the study, the mean consumption was 48.1 units (one unit being equivalent to half a pint of normal-strength beer, lager, cider or stout, a single bar-room measure of spirits, or a glass of wine); 83 per cent of women had smoked cannabis, and a third of women had at some stage used heroin (Morgan Thomas *et al.*, 1990; Plant, 1990; Morgan Thomas *et al.*, 1989). Plant (1997) argues that these high rates can be due to a variety of factors. First, in some locales people engage in sex work to pay for alcohol or drug supplies. Second, the conditions of work and the social milieux surrounding sex work can foster the use of both legal and illicit psychoactive drugs. However, it should be born in mind that the rates of drug use found in Edinburgh may well be unrepresentatively high.

The risk of injury and abuse resulting from client assault is known to be high, especially for street workers. It has even been suggested that prostitution is 'very often about violence' as well as about sex (Barnard, 1993). McKeganey and Barnard (1996) reported that violence against women working the streets of Glasgow was commonplace. However, they do offer a 'cautionary note' to the effect that 'although violence was reported by nearly all of the women interviewed, only a minority of actual encounters between prostitutes and their clients involved violence. Most encounters proceeded in a straightforward way without any untoward occurrence' (McKeganey and Barnard, 1996, p. 70). However, the potential for violence was omnipresent. Women were cynical about police and court commitment and neutrality, and rarely reported attacks (Scutt, 1994). Instead they relied on their own preventive strategies, namely taking control of encounters, relying on intuition born of experience, adopting working rules, working with other women, and carrying weapons.

Perhaps the most neglected of women sex workers' health needs are those general needs which they share with non-sex workers. It is not unreasonable to conjecture that the general health status of sex workers, especially street workers, might be poorer than that of non-sex workers in equivalent age categories. This is first of all because for many of them sex work affords only temporary respite from – or constitutes an 'act of resistance' in the face of – relative poverty (McLeod, 1982) and second because of the unpredictable, stigmatizing and frequently stressful nature of sex work. Both relative poverty and threatening life events are known to underlie poor general health status (and may, too, make sexually transmitted diseases more likely) (Payne, 1991; see also Scambler and Scambler, 1995a).

Limits and limitations of existing care

Service delivery and use

It follows from the discussion above that women sex workers share the same general health needs as others, but also have special needs related to their work (see also Scambler and Scambler, 1995b). There is some evidence that they are likely to be registered with general practitioners (GPs), although they may not disclose their work, thus limiting their freedom to consult openly and their GPs' opportunity to arrange appropriate referrals. This reticence about disclosing their work may be understandable in the light of one national study's finding that 36 per cent of GPs approved of HIV testing for women sex workers without consent, with 75 per cent being willing to share a positive result with practice partners and other physicians, also without consent (Gallagher *et al.*, 1989).

Reluctance to confide fully in GPs and staff in family planning clinics for general as well as special health problems is reflected in the (frequently opportunistic) reliance on tried and tested relationships with health workers in hospital-based clinics. Many problems presented in STD or other specialized clinics, for example, are general, or not related to sex work, and sometimes require referral elsewhere.

'Active' outreach programmes initiated by centres such as the Praed Street Project at St Mary's Hospital in London recognize that neither the general health needs nor the special health needs of women sex workers are currently being satisfied by the often user-unfriendly routine 'passive' primary or secondary services. Need for treatment, care, advice and support is not always translated into demand. Morgan Thomas (1992, pp. 80–1) gives some indication of the wide range of services being developed by active outreach workers in different communities within the UK:

- information on HIV/AIDS and transmission of the virus;
- provision of a range of condoms and prophylactics to cover all sexual services and client groups;
- health services, including screening and treatment where necessary, for sexually transmitted diseases, as well as primary health and dental care;
- drug-related services, including the provision of sterile injecting equipment, education and materials for cleaning equipment, information on safer drug use, access to drug treatment programmes (including maintenance on the drug of choice), medical treatment for drug-related problems, crisis support;
- welfare and legal services, providing information and access to services;
- support through individual and group counselling;
- support in providing facilities for sex workers to meet and discuss issues;
- advocacy for sex workers.

Yet outreach work remains exceptionally difficult, not least because women tend to be apprehensive and wary. The heterogeneity of sex work discussed earlier is relevant here, as an outreach strategy of proven effectiveness for one type of work or locality can fail in another (even different streets within the same red-light district can possess distinctive properties). Central London Action on Street Health (CLASH) has contacted women working from Soho flats and on the streets around King's Cross, but progress has been slow. For example, only one in three of those referred on to statutory services actually attends (Rhodes *et al.*, 1991).

Health promotion

In a discussion of health promotion in relation to the sex industry published elsewhere (Scambler and Scambler, 1995a), we have distinguished between three levels of change, namely 'operational', 'political' and 'structural'.

Operational change refers to health promotion or service initiatives directed by health workers or other experts at the public or at key groups or key settings which neither challenge nor threaten the core social institutions of society. Operational change presents as apolitical and is the easiest level of change to achieve, but its impact is extremely variable.

Political change refers to initiatives which bear on health but are outside the conventional sway of health workers. Ultimately the intervention and sponsorship of government are required. Change at the political level enhances awareness of the core institutions of society and may, typically indirectly, challenge or threaten them.

Structural change refers to fundamental revisions within society's core social institutions which bear on health but which are beyond the capacities of both health workers and parliamentary governments to deliver. Change at the structural level typically requires a mobilization of mass public support which, in turn, typically requires sustained and organized extra-parliamentary political action.

Drawing on these distinctions we have contended that service initiatives and health promotion relevant to women sex workers since the mid-1980s have been restricted almost exclusively to the operational level, and that this is as unproductive in its consequences as it is compatible with UK core social institutions. This is *not in any sense* intended as a criticism of committed health workers. The point is rather that so long as initiatives occur only at the operational level of change, then however commendable and worthwhile they may be, they necessarily amount to little more than exercises in damage limitation (Scambler and Graham-Smith, 1992).

We have proffered a more radical agenda for change under the rubric of health promotion. A summary of our conclusions will suffice here. Our agenda is one which embraces change at all three levels. At the operational level we have argued for a shift in the orientation of health education and prevention programmes in acknowledgement of the fact that sex work involves not only sex workers but also clients, who probably outnumber sex workers by at least 50 to 1, and third parties such as brothel managers, pimps and law enforcement agencies (Morgan Thomas, 1992). In fact there is evidence that many sex workers are already active in health education and prevention, especially in relation to safer sex practices with clients; they should no more be stereotypically cast as passive recipients than they should be deemed to be the sole targets of such programmes (Kinnell, 1989).

At the political level, consideration needs to be given to health education targeted at government agencies. We highlighted two principal objectives. The first is the decriminalization (*not* legalization) of sex work through the abolition of those laws that are specific to prostitution, a reform that is aptly seen as a form of what Downie *et al.* (1990) term 'health protection'. Necessarily linked to any campaign for decriminalization would be a call for the extension of normal citizenship rights to women in the sex industry, ranging from welfare benefits to tax liability.

The second objective concerns an assault, in so far as it is within the capacity of government agencies effectively to sustain one, on the growing phenomenon of relative poverty among women in general and single mothers in particular (Lister, 1992). Such an assault – an example of health protection on a number of accounts – would militate against involuntary recruitment to the sex industry (independently of its legal status).

So far as structural change is concerned, we advocated a greater awareness and a corpus of research-based knowledge of the significance of change at the structural level for the distribution of health. Structural change may, of course, be a precondition for effective political and operational change. In the UK, women's continuing economic and (hierarchic hetero)sexual dependencies are an intrinsic part of a 'system of patriarchal institutions, norms and relationships', as are the constrained, marginal and often health-exacting lives of women sex workers (Scambler *et al.*, 1990). Structural change, too, can constitute a form of health protection.

The concept and politics of empowerment

Rhodes *et al.* (1991) usefully distinguish between four models which inform community-based approaches to health promotion: the *information-giving* or *preventive* model; the *self-empowerment* model; the *community-action* model; and the *radical-political* or *social transformatory model*. Approaches issuing from the information-giving or preventive model employ biomedical definitions of health and illness. They give priority to the imparting of information 'based on the belief that there are causal links between individuals receiving health information messages and modifying their health behaviour' (Rhodes *et al.*, 1991, p. 5). A considerable body of research has in fact shown this belief to be highly problematic. Models of self-empowerment are similarly individualistic in orientation, but are rooted in 'informed choice'. They emphasize developing people's ability to control their own health status through personal growth and self-assertiveness. A key difficulty is the frequent need to go beyond the individualism of self-empowerment in order to address salient social and cultural constraints on health behaviour.

Eschewing the individualism and typically 'top-down' approach of the information-giving or preventive and self-empowerment models, community-action and radical-political or socially transformatory models are characteristically collectivist and 'bottom-up' in orientation. The former aim to enhance health by means of community change arising out of collective action, while the latter go a step further in pursuit of far-reaching social change throughout society. In their introduction to radical-political or socially transformatory models, Rhodes *et al.* note that some organizations related to sex work, such as Red Thread in The Netherlands and COYOTE (Call Off Your Old Tired Ethics) in the USA, have called explicitly for what we earlier defined as political and structural change in recognition of the fact that sex workers have insufficient power or opportunity on their own account to create safer working conditions and to promote safer sex within them, 'because of the contradictions which exist between restrictive and punitive official and legal policy on the one hand, and social reality (the demand for commercial sex) on the other' (Rhodes *et al.*, 1991, p. 8).

Elsewhere, Rhodes (1994) usefully explicates a general notion of 'community empowerment'. He argues that this necessarily involves 'questioning critically the values of those in power', adding that 'in the context of public and community health intervention, this demands questioning the concepts of "healthy" and "unhealthy" and the extent to which marginalized individuals and communities have an equity of "choice" over these values' (Rhodes, 1994, p. 57). Rhodes emphasizes the lack of cohesion and solidarity in many marginalized groups. Moreover, there may well be contradictions between programmes intended to further community empowerment and public health programmes. This is because the new public health 'presumes a rationality of choice-making which makes "healthy" choices the "rational" choices' (Thorogood, 1992). It follows that it 'comprises a political and moral agenda, for it cannot allow empowered wrong choices to be right, healthy or rational' (Rhodes, 1994, pp. 58–9).

This discussion suggests certain general conclusions. First, there are many contexts, such as those involving marginalized groups like sex workers, in which individualistic approaches to empowerment promise little return, and may also function to de-politicize problems. Second, prima facie more promising collectivist approaches may yet be undone by new public health initiatives purporting to represent a wider and overriding general interest. Third, the empowerment of particular groups, conceived individualistically or *qua* collectivities, is an independent but not an absolute principle, that is, it has to be balanced against other – sometimes overriding – principled imperatives.

Civil society and public deliberation

We proffer the view in this concluding section that the nature and extent of the empowerment of women sex workers is a matter for public deliberation in civil society. Our own recommendations for steps to improve the health and well-being of these women clearly presuppose a measure of empowerment contingent on operational and political change, and require the further empowerment of *all women* at both political and structural levels. Self-evidently, however, the case for such empowerment cannot be made solely in the health domain, and much wider issues are involved (see Scambler and Scambler, 1997).

This is not the place for a sustained consideration of the concept of civil society (see Seligman, 1992). It will be sufficient to define it as that *space*, independent of both economy and state, which allows for the possibility of an open and egalitarian consideration of contemporary issues. It is a space characterized by the 'public use of reason'. Following Habermas (1996, p. 367), its core may be said to comprise a network of associations that institutionalizes 'problem-solving discourses on questions of general interest'. Civil society, thus defined, is of course over-shadowed by 'mass media and large agencies, observed by market and opinion research, and inundated by the public relations work, propaganda, and advertising of political parties and groups' (Habermas, 1996, p. 367).

Cobb *et al.* (1976) distinguish usefully between three models of how new issues – like the appropriate nature and extent of the empowerment of women sex workers – emerge and fare:

1. *inside access model* – where the initiative is generated and pursued by office-holders or political leaders, while the broader public is either excluded altogether or able to exercise very little influence;
2. *mobilization model* – where the initiative is again taken within the political system, but where the support of a mobilized public sphere is required to effect change;
3. *outside initiative model* – where it is a mobilized public sphere, or the pressure of public opinion, that promotes an issue to the point of salience and concern in the political system.

Of the outside initiative model, Cobb *et al.* have written:

> The outside initiative model applies to the situation in which a group outside the government structure (1) articulates a grievance, (2) tries to expand interest in the issue to enough other groups in the population to gain a place on the public agenda, in order to (3) create sufficient pressure on decision-makers to force the issue on to the formal agenda for their serious consideration.
>
> This model of agenda-building is likely to predominate in more egalitarian societies. Formal agenda status, however, does not necessarily mean that the final decisions of the authorities or the actual policy implementation will be what the grievance group originally sought.
>
> (Cobb *et al.*, 1976, p. 132)

So far as the empowerment of women in the sex industry is concerned, it is probably campaigns like those mounted by the English Collective of Prostitutes (1997) and its sister groups overseas, most notably for the abolition of the prostitution laws, which have – in line with the outside initiative model – had the most impact. Habermas makes the general point that 'only through their controversial presentation in the media do such topics reach the larger public and subsequently gain a place on the "public agenda"' (Habermas, 1996, p. 381). Protracted campaigning and mass protests, even civil disobedience, he continues, may be required before an issue can progress 'via the surprising election of marginal candidates or radical parties, expanded platforms of "established" parties, important court decisions, and so on, into the core of the political system' (Habermas, 1996, p. 381).

While there is undoubtedly already a public sense of unease in the face of the hypocrisy and ineffectiveness of extant legal statutes, it seems likely that, even if the case for reform was accepted, the demand for decriminalization would be transmuted into some form of legalization or regulationism (Carroll and Scambler, 1996; Scambler and Scambler, 1997).

A 'rethinking' of sex work is certainly long overdue. The challenge remains to achieve this through genuine democratic public deliberation in a revitalized civil society. The focus of such a deliberation, even if triggered by narrower concerns of health, would surely be the gendered links between sex work, politics and social structure.

References

Barbara 1993: 'It's a pleasure doing business with you'. *Social Text* **37**, 11–22.

Barnard, M. 1993: Violence and vulnerability: conditions of work for streetworking prostitutes. *Sociology of Health and Illness* **15**, 683–705.

Barton, S., Taylor-Robinson, D. and Harris, J. 1987: Female prostitutes and sexually transmitted diseases. *British Journal of Hospital Medicine* **7**, 34–45.

Boyle, S. 1994: *Working girls and their men: male sexual desires and fantasies revealed by the women paid to satisfy them.* London: Smith Gryphon Ltd.

Brittan, A. 1989: *Masculinity and power.* Oxford: Basil Blackwell.

Carroll, N. and Scambler, G. 1996: Public attitudes towards women sex workers against the background of the AIDS epidemic. Working Paper 2. London: Unit of Medical Sociology, University College London.

Cobb, R., Ross, J. and Ross, M. 1976: Agenda building as a comparative political process. *American Political Science Review* **70**, 126–38.

Davies, P. and Feldman, R. 1997: Prostitute men now. In Scambler, G. and Scambler, A. (eds), *Rethinking prostitution: purchasing sex in the 1990s.* London: Routledge, 29–53.

Day, S., Ward, H., Wadsworth, J. and Harris, J. 1987: Attitudes to barrier protection among female prostitutes in London. Unpublished paper.

Day, S., Ward, H. and Harris, J. 1988: Prostitute women and public health. *British Medical Journal* **297**, 1585.

Downie, R., Fyfe, C. and Tannahill, A. 1990: *Health promotion: models and values*. Oxford: Oxford Medical Publications.

English Collective of Prostitutes (1997) Campaigning for legal change. In Scambler, G. and Scambler, A. (eds), *Rethinking prostitution: purchasing sex in the 1990s*. London: Routledge, 83–102.

European Working Group on HIV Infection in Female Prostitutes (EWGHFP) 1993: HIV in European female sex workers: epidemiological link with use of petroleum-based lubricants. *AIDS* 7, 401–8.

French, D. 1988: *Working: my life as a prostitute*. London: Gollancz.

Gallagher, M., Rhodes, T., Foy, C. *et al*. 1989: *A national study of HIV infection, AIDS and general practice*. Health Care Research Unit, Report No. 36. Newcastle upon Tyne: University of Newcastle upon Tyne.

Giddens, A. 1992: *The transformation of intimacy: sexuality, love and eroticism in modern society*. Cambridge: Polity Press.

Habermas, J. 1996: *Between facts and norms: contributions to a discourse theory of law and democracy*. Cambridge: Polity Press.

Kinnell, H. 1989: *Prostitutes, their clients and risks of HIV infection in Birmingham*. Occasional paper. Birmingham: Department of Public Health Medicine.

Lister, R. 1992: *Women's economic dependency and social security*. Manchester: Equal Opportunities Commission.

McKeganey, N. and Barnard, M. 1996: *Sex work on the streets: prostitutes and their clients*. Buckingham: Open University Press.

McKeganey, N., Barnard, M., Leyland, A., Coote, I. and Follet, E. 1992: Female street-working prostitution and HIV infection in Glasgow. *British Medical Journal* 305, 801–4.

McLeod, E. 1982: *Working women: prostitution now*. London: Croom-Helm.

Morgan Thomas, R. 1992: HIV and the sex industry. In Bury, J., Morrison, V. and Mclachlan, S. (eds), *Working with women and AIDS: medical, social and counselling issues*. London: Routledge, 71–84.

Morgan Thomas, R., Plant, M., Plant, M. and Sales, J. 1990: Risk of HIV infection among clients of the sex industry in Scotland. *British Medical Journal* 301, 525.

Morgan Thomas, R., Plant, M.A., Plant, M.L., and Sales, D.I. 1989: Risk of AIDS among workers in the sex industry: some initial results from a Scottish study. *British Medical Journal* 299, 148–9.

Naffine, N. 1987: *Female crime: the construction of women in criminology*. London: Allen & Unwin.

O'Neill, M. 1997: Prostitute women now. In Scambler, G. and Scambler, A. (eds), *Rethinking prostitution: purchasing sex in the 1990s*. London: Routledge, 3–28.

Payne, S. 1991: *Women, health and poverty*. London: Harvester Wheatsheaf.

Perkins, R. and Bennett, G. 1985: *Being a prostitute: prostitute women and prostitute men*. Sydney: Allen & Unwin.

Pheterson, G. 1993: The whore stigma: female dishonour and male unworthiness. *Social Text* 37, 39–54.

Plant, M. 1990: *AIDS, drugs and prostitution*. London: Routledge.

Plant, M. 1997: Alcohol, drugs and social milieu. In Scambler, G. and Scambler, A. (eds), *Rethinking prostitution: purchasing sex in the 1990s*. London: Routledge, 164–79.

Rhodes, T. 1994: Outreach, community change and community empowerment: contradictions for public health and health promotion. In Aggleton, P., Davies, P. and Hart, G. (eds), *AIDS: foundations for the future*. London: Taylor & Francis, 48–64.

Rhodes, T., Holland, J. and Hartnoll, R. 1991: *Hard to reach or out of reach? An evaluation of an innovative model of HIV outreach health education*. London: Tufnell Press.

Scambler, G. 1997: Conspicuous and inconspicuous sex work: the neglect of the ordinary and mundane. In Scambler, G. and Scambler, A. (eds), *Rethinking prostitution: purchasing sex in the 1990s*. London: Routledge, 105–20.

Scambler, G. and Graham-Smith, R. 1992: Female prostitution and AIDS: the realities of social exclusion. In Aggleton, P., Davies, P. and Hart, G. (eds), *AIDS: rights, risk and reason*. London: Falmer Press, 68–76.

Scambler, G. and Scambler, A. 1995a: Social change and health promotion among women sex workers in London. *Health Promotion International* **10**, 17–24.

Scambler, G. and Scambler, A. 1995b: *Health issues for women and men sex workers in London. Final Report*. London: King's Fund.

Scambler, G. and Scambler, A. 1997: Afterword: rethinking prostitution. In Scambler, G. and Scambler, A. (eds), *Rethinking prostitution: purchasing sex in the 1990s*. London: Routledge, 180–8.

Scambler, G., Peswani, R., Renton, A. and Scambler, A. 1990: Women prostitutes in the AIDS era. *Sociology of Health and Illness* **12**, 260–73.

Scutt, J. 1994: Judicial vision – rape, prostitution and the chaste woman. *Women's Studies International Forum* **17**, 345–56.

Seligman, A. 1992: *The idea of civil society*. New York: The Free Press.

Silver, R. 1993: *The girl in scarlet heels*. London: Century.

Thorogood, N. 1992: What is the relevance of sociology for health promotion? In Bunton, R. and MacDonald, G. (eds), *Health promotion: disciplines and diversity*. London: Routledge, 42–65.

Ward, H. and Day, S. 1997: Health care and regulation: new perspectives. In Scambler, G. and Scambler, A. (eds) *Rethinking prostitution: selling sex in the 1990s*. London: Routledge, 139–63.

Ward, H., Day, S., Mezzone, J. *et al*. 1993: Prostitution and risk of HIV: female prostitutes in London. *British Medical Journal* **307**, 356–8.

Woolley, P., Bowman, C. and Kinghorn, G. 1988: Prostitution in Sheffield: differences between prostitutes. *Genito-urinary Medicine* **64**, 391–3.

6

Empowering communities: the case of childhood accidents

Helen Roberts[6.1]

What could be less empowering than the death of a child? What could be more painful for a parent than living in a community where one's child is at risk?

This chapter describes the extent of the child accident problem and some of the traditional policy and practice responses. It then goes on to look at three case studies. The first is in Corkerhill, a former railway village and now a community marked by disadvantage in Glasgow. The second is based on a school community in inner-city Glasgow. The third case study is based on Wardleworth, a community in Rochdale, with a substantial ethnic minority population. All three of these communities developed robust strategies in relation to accident prevention, in tandem with research projects.

The chapter goes on to look at the World Health Organization's Safe Community network, and finally examines the concept of 'empowerment' and the extent to which it can be made meaningful in research and practice around child accidents.

Introduction

Injuries are the main cause of death to children in the UK (Woodroffe *et al.*, 1993). Moreover, they make a considerable contribution to childhood morbidity (ill health) and the use of hospital beds. Dangers in the home and the wider community are a source of anxiety to parents, and thus the impact of risks and dangers on the well-being of children and adults is formidable.

Child accidents: the extent of the problem

First, a word on the language used in this chapter. Child accidents are not just a health problem. They also constitute a problem for those managing environmental, transport and leisure and social services. Not all child accidents lead to injury, but the *risk* of child accidents – irrespective of whether there is a direct health effect – leads to indirect health effects, and a restriction on the freedom which children have to explore their worlds (Hillman *et al.*, 1990). For this reason, while the preferred term in medical circles for this area of work is 'injuries' (i.e. the sequelae, or what follows accidents) I refer more usually to accidents and risk (i.e. the antecedents or what happens before the injury). It is in looking at changing these antecedents that we can most effectively work with communities. This is not to underplay the enormous effect which improved tertiary care in specialized hospital units has had on accident survival for children. Indeed, there is some informed speculation that it is the combination of improved hospital care and increased surveillance and self-surveillance of children (resulting in a restriction in their healthy capacity to learn through exploration) that accounts for the drop in child injury deaths.

While childhood cancers (leukaemia in particular) and childhood health problems such as asthma and other respiratory disorders have a relatively high public profile, child accidents are a less prominent issue on the public health and social policy agenda (Roberts and Roberts, 1997). This is despite the fact that deaths from unintended injury are the main cause of death in children over the age of 1 year in the UK.

Moreover, the social class gradient in child accident deaths, i.e. the gap between those from the most and least advantaged backgrounds, is steeper than for any other cause of death. Poverty damages children's health, and nowhere is this clearer than in the example of child accidents. Poorer children are up to 15 times more likely to die in a house fire than children from a more economically advantaged background. In addition, they are more likely to die on the road or in a home accident. While there has been some overall reduction in the number of child accident deaths in recent years, the gap between rich and poor children actually *widened* between 1981 and 1991 (Roberts and Power, 1996).

The social patterning of childhood injuries and death belies the common view that accidents are random, unpredictable events. Child accidents demonstrate clear social, regional and gender patterns (Avery *et al.*, 1990; Roberts *et al.*, 1996). They are more likely to occur at particular times of day (the time when children are returning from school) and at particular times of year. Some areas of the UK (those most characterized by economic and social disadvantage) have higher child injury rates than others. Boys are at greater risk from injury than girls. This social patterning should give us pointers about causality, and these in turn should aid us in the development of effective strategies for accident prevention.

Policy and practice responses to child accidents

With the exception of accidents where a number of children are involved – minibus accidents and recreational and school journey accidents are cases in point – policy responses to the problem of child accidents are fragmented and poorly co-ordinated. The problem of child accidents crosses the areas of responsibility of a number of government and local authority departments. In that sense, accidents are nobody's baby. While *The Health of the Nation* (Department of Health, 1992) targeted a reduction of 33 per cent in the death rate from accidents to under-15s in England and Wales by the year 2005, the means suggested for bringing about this reduction were mainly restricted to educational initiatives whose effectiveness is largely unproven (Towner *et al.,* 1993). *First Steps for the NHS,* for instance (National Health Service Management Executive, 1992), advocates the provision of health promotion material on accident prevention in community-based clinics and other appropriate locations, while the White Paper itself signalled that the government intended to rely primarily on information and education for the prevention of accidents 'and to avoid the imposition of unneccessary regulations on business and individuals' (Department of Health, 1992, p. 106). The green paper *Our Healthier Nation* (Department of Health, 1998) again singled out accidents as a national priority, acknowledging the widening gap in inequalities in health.

Accidents are one of those areas of health where prevention has a number of attractions other than the obvious one. As Stone (1989, p. 891) has pointed out: 'health education is cheap, generally uncontroversial and safe: if it works, politicians take the credit, and if it does not, the target population takes the blame.' Much of the practice response has been to 'target' the education or re-education of parents and children. The victims of accidents are thus educated to take avoidance behaviour.

The flaws in this approach are clear. Take a simple example. Children are exhorted not to cross the road when a car is coming, and not to cross between parked cars. How realistic is this in the urban environments which most of them inhabit (Thomson, 1996)?

To take another example, a safety organization suggests that accidents happen to children who are over-protected, under-protected, angry, tired or showing off. They are more likely to happen when adults are under stress or less alert. It is suggested that risks can be reduced by making sure that the home and garden are as safe as possible, never leaving children on their own, and buying toys and equipment that are safety approved and checked. This is well-meaning enough advice, no doubt, but what might it entail *in practice*? What do you do if you are a Glaswegian mother living three flights up, with three children, and you need to hang your washing on the green ? Do you leave your children alone, or do you take all three of them down 72 stone steps with you? How are risks balanced in everyday life? Are instructions not to leave your children unattended likely to reduce the risk to them, or might these messages themselves promote poor health since, while doing nothing to reduce the level of childhood risk, they increase the level of parental anxiety? As we shall see from the case studies below, what is extraordinary about child accidents, given the unsafe environments in which most children spend most of their lives, is not that they happen, but that children survive to adulthood at all. Childhood and parenthood increasingly involve complex risk avoidance strategies. Given this, it makes sense that the well-informed health worker should understand that they have a good deal to learn from those who negotiate unsafe environments daily.

Case study examples of community involvement in safety

The principles of a community approach to a problem involve the participation in and ownership of agendas by all involved, and particularly those on the receiving end of health promotion interventions. Traditional methods of health education use a more directive, top-down approach. The experts define the problem, and then suggest solutions.

All three case studies described below draw on a common approach, that is, research based on the principle that people are experts on their own environments, and they develop strategies – often rather effective ones – for managing this risk. People, including children, have reservoirs of knowledge on which we as 'experts' can draw, if we listen to them.

Case study one – Safety as a social value: Corkerhill

An area of high risk for children, typical of many throughout the UK, is Corkerhill, a community of some 2000 people in the south of Glasgow. It is bordered on one side by a river, on another by a busy main road, and on a third by a railway line – the site of a recent child death. However, to one side of the community is a beautiful stretch of open land, Pollock Park, which houses the Burrell art collection, left to the people of Glasgow. In the last few years the community has been effectively cut off from easy access to this open land by the construction of a new motorway, which was fiercely resisted by local people, who have a low rate of car ownership.

The community is characterized by an accident rate which is twice the city average, high unemployment, a high level of local authority housing, few local leisure facilities and generally poor housing stock. These paint a depressingly familiar picture. However, the place is also characterized by a strong community spirit, a strong desire to see children flourish, and a strong willingness to do everything that can be done to achieve this.

From 1990 to 1992, the community was the location for a piece of research looking at safety as a social value, exploring the ways in which parents keep their children safe in an unsafe environment (Roberts, 1991; Roberts *et al.*, 1992a, 1993, 1995; Rice *et al.*, 1994). The research consisted of three parts.

First, a series of group interviews was conducted with parents from different housing types, and a group of teenagers. These interviews took place over two to three sessions, and were intended to look at the salience that child safety issues had for this particular community, given that it was only one aspect of a seamless web of difficulties, insecurities and health risks faced by the community. In the first week, we explored issues ranging from what people think about when they hear others talking about an accident, to the types of accident that are common in Corkerhill, and accidents which nearly but did not quite happen. In the second week, we explored features of the home which promoted safety, and those which put children at risk, the features outside the home which put children at risk, and the most dangerous places in Corkerhill. In the third week, we looked at the extent to which people worried about accidents, and what the consequences of this worry were. Finally, we looked at what might be done to make things safer with an unlimited budget, a budget able to tackle only two or three problems, and with no budget, but the power to change the way in which existing services are organized. The unlimited budget option brought calls for the housing to be completely rebuilt, with gardens, and for there to be a full review of traffic, with traffic-calming measures. One person drew a detailed plan of how this might work. A budget able to tackle two or three problems would again deal with the built environment, including changes to housing, attention to problems with the windows, and traffic-calming measures. Service provision, such as adequate day care for children, was also mentioned. The no-cost options also involved day care and child care, on a reciprocal or neighbourhood basis, reorganizing the times at which the rubbish bins were collected, and better systems for ensuring that local workmen ensured safety. (In contrast, a group of professionals asked similar questions came up with very dissimilar answers, with the overwhelming emphasis on safety education for parents and children.)

Second, a survey of every household in the community – in effect a census – questioned those who lived in the community on issues ranging from the extent of adult anxiety to the number and type of accidents per child. It is perhaps a measure of the close 'fit' between the researchers' agenda and that of the community that the response rate for the survey was 95 per cent for households with a child aged 14 years or under, and 84 per cent for other households in the community. We found that, moreover, just under half (46 per cent) of Corkerhill's families had experienced one or more serious childhood accidents in the study year, the majority of parents worry most of the time that their children might be involved in an accident while at home, in the street or at school. Four in five parents worry about the safety of children in the street, and over half worry about their safety in the home and at school. In total, over three-quarters of parents (76 per cent) think that Corkerhill is very unsafe for children.

Third, we conducted a series of case studies of accidents, near-accidents and averted accidents identified through the survey. Much of the data currently collected on accidents is hospital based. This means that we have more data on the sequelae of accidents – injuries – than on their antecedents. What was it that led to the accident? What might have averted it? Data on near-accidents are commonplace in high-risk activities such as aviation and anaesthetics. Examining these data in a 'no blame' context is one means of averting in future those accidents which did not quite happen this time round. While many children benefit at an individual level from this approach ('I did this last time, and that scary thing happened, so I'll avoid it in future'), we do little to systematize these data and learn from them. We collected data on 12 near-accidents. One, for instance, involved a toddler almost falling from a window which she had accidentally opened by knocking the handle. This was reported to the appropriate authorities: 'I said that the windows could be easily opened, and they said they didn't have the money. So they are still the same.' Another parent told us: 'We had about a year when the putty hadn't set in the window.' Most parents felt that it was primarily good luck that prevented near-accidents from becoming real injuries, although in almost every case there is evidence that what really happened was a consequence of quick thinking and swift action on the part of one or more adults, or the children themselves (Roberts *et al.*, 1995).

The Corkerhill project was not an action research project. It had no preventive component as such, but it ran alongside preventive efforts in the community. The group interviews acted as one focus for collective concern, and ultimately for collective action. Initiatives stemming from the period when this work was carried out include a new playgroup ('The Wee Horrors'), a scheme enabling children in the community to mark and label sources of danger, and an active (although ultimately unsuccessful) campaign against the building of a new motorway only yards from some of the houses in Corkerhill.

Other indirect gains have been an increase in the already considerable expertise of people living in the community, some of whom acted as paid community consultants to the project. They spoke about the project on national and local radio and television, a television programme on keeping children safe was made in the community, two community members went to a world congress on safe communities in Atlanta, Georgia, to share their experiences and knowledge, and one person got a job with a nearby safe community project. The community became part of the world-wide network of Safe Communities.

Whether it actually became a safe – or safer – community is another matter. The extent to which the work in the community could be considered empowering will be discussed below, in tandem with the other two case studies.

Case study two – Child accidents in an inner-city primary school

Hillhead Primary is an inner-city, multi-ethnic primary school of some 500 children in Glasgow. It is a Victorian school, built on several levels, with three small playgrounds.

At the time that a raft of child accident research in the unit where I was then employed was being carried out, it struck me as odd that, while there is a whole field dedicated to work-related accidents for adults, there is very little research looking at accidents which happen to children in their workplaces – schools, or on the journey to and from school (Roberts, 1996). We aimed to find a means of working productively with children in the school, including the youngest children, on their perspectives on school safety, and their strategies for reducing risk and making schools a safer place (Roberts *et al.*, 1992b, 1993; Roberts, 1996a,b).

Our strategy was as follows. The youngest children were encouraged to describe safe and unsafe places in the school, or on the journey to or from school, and to draw these, or to draw accidents they had seen. Older children were given a similar exercise, but were also shown epidemiological data we had collected on school accidents right across Glasgow. These data described accidents categorized according to time, place, activity and injury. They further described the age and sex of the child involved, and the location of the school was taken as a proxy for social class. We asked the children to whom we showed the data – which were displayed as bar charts and pie charts – to suggest what they meant. Why did so many more boys than girls have accidents? Why did relatively few accidents happen in relatively dangerous places, such as school laboratories? Why were there peaks at certain times in the school day? Why were there many accidents in primary school playgrounds, but few in the playgrounds of secondary schools? The children could have *been* epidemiologists. They were sophisticated in their understanding of what could, and could not, be drawn from these statistical data. They drew our attention to the influence of reporting bias. They understood that rules in laboratories probably made them safer, and that while primary school playgrounds involve a lot of rushing around, secondary school playgrounds involve hanging out and looking cool.

Why do older children have more accidents than younger ones?

Responses included the following.

> '*Wee ones don't play such rough games.*'
> '*Wee ones just sit around and cuddle each other.*'
> '*Bigger ones have more fun.*'

Why do boys have more accidents than girls?

Responses included the following.

> '*Girls fight less.*'
> '*Girls are more sensible.*'
> '*Some boys just want to have accidents to prove how macho they are. They get their head split open, then just say "ow".*'

In relation to their own school community, we asked children how they might make the school a safer place. We asked them to describe their journeys to and from school, and to mark with a skull and crossbones the areas which they considered to be dangerous. We asked them to redesign their school playground, and to devise 'rules' for a safer school. These included the following.

'Don't trip people up or hurt them.'
'No smoking staff ! Because I have asthma.'

Other ideas included the following.

'Painting the edges of the stairs.'
'Remove the spiky railings.'
'Putting benches in the playground.'

Ideas for making the playground safer included the following.

'A quiet corner.'
'A first aid area.'
'Some resting and fasting areas.'
'A corner for getting the things you might need for playing your games.'

As can be seen from the children's responses, they perceive their health and safety in a holistic way. Health (my asthma), religious and cultural observances (fasting) and remedial action (a first aid area) are all part of the children's overall vision.

We showed the children what could be done with data kept in the school's own accident book, and how details of accidents recorded there might teach us how to prevent similar events in the future. We made a video with the children, describing their approach to school safety, and including the worksheets the Hillhead children had helped us to devise and use (Roberts and University of Glasgow Media Services, 1992).

Meanwhile, parents mobilized around the school safety issue liaised with the local police and roads department about traffic congestion around the school, attempted to tackle some aspects of school fire safety, and organized some painting to improve the environment of the children's play areas and encourage non-combat games.

Were the children empowered? Did the accident rate in the school drop? The answer to the first question is that the children seemed to enjoy being consulted about their own environments, and exercised an admirable degree of judgement and wisdom in their responses. Children have a strong sense of what is fair and what is not, and particularly relished telling us about the misdeeds of car drivers along the Great Western Road which skirts their school:

'It was the time I was walking to school, and the green man was on, and I was walking across, and this car went straight through the green man, and I just moved back in time, otherwise I would have been knocked down.'

Children had sensible strategies, and some of these were put into effect by the school. There was some staggering of playtimes, and some 'sharing' of play space between those who did and those who did not want to use the entire play area for Scotland's favourite sport. An informal monitoring system was used to help curb bullying, and to discourage fights.

Case study three – Child accident prevention in Wardleworth: Rochdale

The final example is rather different to the first two. In the case of Corkerhill, the work done resulted from a combination of researcher interest and community drive. In the second case, the work was a combination of an academic interest in the risks in the child's workplace (school), and maternal anxiety (mine) about the level of incidents – accidents or bullying – in my (then) 7-year-old's school.

In the case of Wardleworth, a group of highly motivated professionals wanted to do something about the level of child accidents in Wardleworth, an area of Rochdale, and wanted to use similar methods to those we had tried in Glasgow – that is, to draw on the reservoir of knowledge in the community to identify unsafe places and practices, and to involve the community in strategies to reduce risks. The Child Accident Prevention Group in Rochdale commissioned a piece of research, and Barnardo's made a successful tender to carry out the work.

In carrying out the study, we worked with parents and professionals in the community, and with a local school in much the same way as we had in Glasgow, and on the basis of this we were able to make a number of recommendations directed at specific sections of local government (McNeish *et al.*, 1996).

Even where there are play areas, children and their families may be reluctant to use them. The children in our Wardleworth survey gave some reasons why:

'The place is full of dog poo.' (Parveen, Wardleworth)
'It is far from our house.' (Rehana, Wardleworth)
'There might be dangerous things in it.' (Mohammed, Wardleworth)
'Sometimes, I'm not allowed to play out.' (Firoz, Wardleworth)

As part of our work in Wardleworth, we asked a group of primary school children to monitor the traffic lights on the level crossing outside their school. The crossing has an on-site lollipop man. Did any cars go through on a red light? They did. Over a period of 1 hour, the children counted 31 cars going through the lights on red, and a further 73 cars going through on amber. Was the lollipop man surprised? No he was not. 'This is not unusual. I regularly nearly get run over' (McNeish and Roberts, 1995, p. 19).

Children were among the groups who came up with recommendations for the council:

'Someone to watch the playground and look after us.'
'Soft floors in playgrounds.'

They were well aware of the dangers of local roads:

'Put ramps on the road to slow down the cars and other vehicles.'
'Make a bridge going over the road.'

One lad felt that a sterner approach was needed:

'Police walking round with bulletproof jackets and guns.'

The recommendations of children and other interest groups were discussed with the relevant professionals at a one-day meeting, and they identified action points. What is perhaps most outstanding about Rochdale's approach is that the Children's Plan there has been informed by, and is responsive to, the areas of safety identified by children and parents. 'Child protection' is not seen only in terms of the safety of children within the private domain of the family, but public responsibility is taken for dangers in the wider environment.

The Safe Community Network

The Safe Community Network, co-ordinated by the Department of Social Medicine at the Karolinska Institute in Stockholm,[62] aims to bring together communities with common interests to reduce or prevent injuries. Those communities which become members are not necessarily 'safe', – but have aspirations to become safer and to share lessons learned with other communities world-wide. Communities which are part of the movement include Corkerhill (Morrison *et al.*, 1992), in Glasgow, various municipalities in the Nordic countries, and communities in regions as diverse as India and South Africa.

Those who wish to participate in the network need to demonstrate the following:

- the existence of a cross-sectoral group responsible for injury prevention;
- involvement of the local community network;
- a programme covering all ages, environments and situations;
- concern for high-risk groups and high-risk environments, and particularly to aim to ensure justice for vulnerable groups;
- those responsible must be able to document the frequency and cause of injuries;
- the programme must be long term.

The community must also undertake to:

- utilize appropriate indicators to evaluate processes and the effects of change;
- analyse the community's organizations and the possibility of their participation in the programme;

- involve health care organizations in both the registration of injuries and the prevention programme;
- be prepared to involve all levels of the community in solving the injury problem;
- disseminate experiences both nationally and internationally;
- be prepared to contribute to a strong network of Safe Communities.

Corkerhill's 18-page application, published by the Karolinska Institute (Morrison *et al.*, 1992), demonstrated a commitment to all of the above 12 indicators, and described Corkerhill's work in these areas. Five years on, the community continues to work with these principles and to support, and be supported by, the Safe Communities network. The work remains voluntary, and is carried out by local people.

To what extent can or does the movement make a difference? As Walter Morrison, the secretary of Corkerhill Community Council, put it: 'We don't just want a certificate on the wall.' A network does not solve the problem of accidents and injuries, but it is one more means by which those wanting to effect change can get together and try to do so.

Empowering communities to make them safe: a useful concept?

There are some things which only local and central government can do to make communities safe – and these things are truly empowering for communities. The provision of safe houses, secure play spaces, adequate day care so that parents (more usually mothers, in practice) have respite from 24-hour child care, the prioritization of children over cars, and taking into account the needs of child pedestrians making the journeys to and from school when setting British summertime – all of these are empowering measures.

What is extraordinary, given the intrinsic lack of safety in our urban environments, is not that there are so *many* accidents, but that there are so *few*. The fact that so many children and families do manage to negotiate dangerous environments successfully indicates that we have a good deal to learn from them in terms of safety strategies. However, in doing so we need to recognize that this safety is bought at a cost, and that this cost entails a restriction on children's freedom to explore their environments. Chronic parental anxiety is a further cost.

As Walter Morrison has suggested: 'If child accidents were contagious, they'd do something about them tomorrow.' Child accidents are a public health problem which can (largely) be localized, and to that extent, to suggest that matters be put right by the efforts of those living in the affected communities can be used as a cynical abrogation of responsibility by those who really do have the power to make changes. The extent to which people who are anxious find it difficult to keep their children safe was confirmed in our work:

> *In order to keep the kids safe, you keep them trapped in the house, you're trapped in the house, you're under more pressure and that in itself is a cause of accidents. If you're going about there like this up to here wi' it, you're no watching your kids, and in that space of time, something happens.*
>
> *You can get really depressed, and think about all the things* [safety equipment] *that your children should have ... and add that to all the other stresses you've got – living in bad housing or poverty and you can get depressed and distracted and that's when accidents are more likely to happen.*

Whether in the three case studies outlined above the communities involved were 'empowered' is open to question. However, we can be more confident that the reservoirs of expert knowledge held by children and parents greatly enriched the knowledge generation in the projects described, and that this in turn had an effect on the community.

Endnotes

6.1. Helen Roberts is Co-ordinator, Research and Development, with the children's charity Barnado's, writing in a personal capacity. Her most recent book on child safety is *Children at risk: safety as a social value*, written with Susan J. Smith and Carol Bryce (Open University Books, 1995). Her interest in this area stems from her observation as a mother that life isn't fair for children. Cars are given priority over children, houses are designed with grown people in mind, and play spaces are much reduced from the time when she was a child (not all that long ago).

6.2. The WHO collaborating centre of community safety promotion is based at the Karolinska Institute, Department of Social Medicine, Kronan Health Centre, S-172 83 Sundbyberg, Sweden.

References

Avery, J.G., Vaudin, J.N., Fletcher, J.L. and Watson, J.M. 1990: Geographical and social variations in mortality due to childhood accidents in England and Wales 1975–1984. *Public Health* **104**, 171–82

Department of Health 1992: *The Health of the Nation: a strategy for health in England.* London: HMSO.

Department of Health 1998: *Our Healthier Nation: a contract for health.* London: HMSO.

Hillman, M., Adams, J., and Whitelegg, J. 1990: *One false move ... a study of children's independent mobility.* London: Policy Studies Institute.

McNeish, D. and Roberts, H. 1995: *Playing it safe.* Barkingside: Barnardo's.

McNeish, D., Roberts, H. and Barrett, A. 1995: *The prevention of child accidents in Wardleworth, Rochdale.* Barkingside: Barnardo's.

Morrison, W., Rice, C., Roberts, H. and Svanstrom, L. 1992: *Corkerhill, Glasgow: application to become a member of the safe community network. Paper no. 275.* Stockholm: Karolinska Institute, Department of Social Medicine.

National Health Service Management Executive 1992: *The Health of the Nation: first steps for the NHS*. London: Department of Health.

Pharaoh, P. and Alberman, E. 1990: Annual statistical review. *Archives of Disease in Childhood* **65**, 147–51.

Rice, C., Roberts, H., Smith, S.J. and Bryce, C. 1994: *It's like teaching your child to swim in a pool full of alligators*. In Popay, J. and Williams, G. (eds), *Researching the people's health*. London: Routledge, 184–200.

Roberts, H. 1991: Accident prevention: a community approach. *Health Visitor* **64**, 219–21.

Roberts, H. 1996a: *Child accidents at home school and play*. In Gillham, W. and Thomson, J. (eds), *Child safety: problems and prevention from pre-school to adolescence*. London: Routledge, 40–54.

Roberts, H. 1996b: *Intervening to prevent accidents: keeping children at safe at home, school and play*. In Gillham, W. and Thomson, J. (eds), *Child safety: problems and prevention from pre-school to adolescence*. London: Routledge, 55–66.

Roberts, H. and University of Glasgow Media Services 1992: *A Safe School is no Accident*. Glasgow: University of Glasgow.

Roberts, H. and Roberts, I. 1997: Poor excuse for neglect. *The Guardian*, Society Supplement 1 January, 18–19.

Roberts, H., Smith, S.J. and Lloyd, M. 1992a: Accident prevention: a public health approach. In Scott, S., Williams, G., Platt, S. and Thomas, H. (eds), *Private risks and public dangers*. Aldershot: Avebury, 184–200.

Roberts, H., Bradby, H. and Kelly, T. 1992b: Safe schools are no accident. *Streetwise, Quarterly Bulletin for the National Association for Urban Studies* **Issue 12**, 12–13.

Roberts, H., Smith, S.J. and Bryce, C. 1993: Prevention is better . . . *Sociology of Health and Illness* **15**, 447–63.

Roberts, H., Smith, S.J. and Bryce C. 1995: *Children at risk: safety as social value*. Buckingham: Open University Press.

Roberts, I. 1996: Safely to school *Lancet* **347**, 1642.

Roberts, I. and Power, C. 1996: Does the decline in child injury mortality vary by social class? A comparison of class-specific mortality in 1981 and 1991. *British Medical Journal* **313**, 784–6.

Roberts, I., Norton, R. and Tauer, B. 1996: The importance of socio-economic and ethnic differences in exposure to risk. *Journal of Epidemiology and Community Health* **50**, 162–5.

Stone, D. 1989: Upside-down prevention. *Health Service Journal* **99**, 890–1.

Thomson, J.A. 1996: Child pedestrian accidents: what makes children vulnerable? In Gillham, W. and Thomson, J.A. (eds), *Child safety: problem and prevention from pre-school to adolescence*. London: Routledge, 67–85.

Towner, E., Dowswell, T. and Jarvis, S. 1993: *The effectiveness of health promotion interventions in the prevention of unintentional childhood injury: a review of the literature*. HEA Policy Review. London: Health Education Authority.

Woodroffe, C., Glickman, M., Barker, M. and Power, C. 1993: *Children, teenagers and health, the key data*. Buckingham: Open University Press.

7

Empowering children through ethnography?

Felicity Hepper, Sally Kendall and Ian Robinson

Introduction

The concept of empowerment in health has been considered from a number of perspectives in this volume. Whilst consideration has been given to both ways in which people could (or indeed should) be empowered and the potential outcomes of this process, a further dimension to this debate concerns the possible ways in which the *research process* may in itself have an empowering effect. The purpose of this chapter is therefore to give due consideration to the question of whether ethnography, as one approach to research, could have an empowering effect on children of primary school age. This immediately poses the question of the position of children in society and their interrelationships with the adult world. It also introduces the notion of children characterized as participants and interactive in research – researching with, rather than researching on. The ways in which children construct their own world, especially in relation to health and illness, were explored by the authors in a study of childhood asthma and its management within a primary school environment. The process of undertaking the research and some case study data which emerged from it will be drawn on to illuminate arguments about the way in which ethnographic data could be utilized to inform policy and practice in relation to child health from the child's perspective.

Ethnography as a source of evidence for health care

According to Hammersley and Atkinson, ethnography 'involves the ethnographer participating, overtly or covertly, in people's daily lives for an extended period of time, watching what happens, listening to what is said, asking questions – in fact, collecting whatever data are available to throw light on the issues which are the focus of the research' (Hammersley and Atkinson, 1995, p.1).

This approach to understanding the social world has long been adopted by anthropologists in order to provide rich descriptions and theoretical positions on cultural differences and diversity. More recently, researchers interested in issues surrounding health in different subgroups have tended to reject the social survey in favour of research designs which provide a more naturalistic account of the ways in which people and groups of people construct their own world. The use of ethnography – often, it would seem, defined in the broadest terms – appears to have become the approach of choice for some health researchers. The apparent shift in medical sociology, and what could loosely be described as health services research, from a more positivist stance on analysing issues of health and illness, to what has been described as a post-positivist (e.g. Lincoln and Guba, 1985) interpretation, may be explained by the realization that logical empiricism does not adequately explain or even predict the natural world of human interaction. There have been many full accounts of the philosophical debate underlying this seemingly simplistic statement (see, for example, Lincoln and Guba, 1985; Carr and Kemmis, 1986; Lather, 1994), and it is not appropriate in this chapter to recycle these arguments. Nevertheless, an important consideration for health researchers is the emphasis which is currently placed on the notion of evidence-based practice.

Sackett *et al.* have defined evidence-based medicine as:

> the conscientious, explicit and judicious use of current best evidence in making decisions about the care of individual patients. The practice of evidence-based medicine means integrating individual clinical expertise with the best available external evidence from systematic research.
>
> (Sackett *et al.*, 1996, p. 71)

Given that most health care involves interaction with people who have their own lay beliefs and explanatory models about health and illness (Kleinman *et al.*, 1978), how do practitioners decide what is the best available evidence? What is the *truth* about the best health care and clinical effectiveness? What is perceived to be effective care medically may be interpreted in a different way by the recipient of care. An example here is non-compliance with medical treatment when the side-effects experienced are worse than the symptoms of the disease itself.

Fairly obviously we cannot assume one interpretation of the truth – philosophers have argued from Socrates to the present day about the nature of the world we live in and the existence of man and womankind within it. However, there does appear to be a trend within the current NHS policy (National Health Service Executive, 1996) to accept quantitative evidence as being closer to the truth about effective care than other forms, this being the randomized controlled trial (RCT). This approach draws upon the experimental method to establish truths about effective health care. Based as it is on logical empiricism, the approach claims to be objective and can take no account of human responses or interaction.

This approach to scientific truth is part of our lives – you only have to witness how it is drawn upon (totally irreverently) in washing powder advertisements, pet food promotions, and so on. However, as Popper (1959) argues, we should never accept even these apparently well-established facts as static knowledge; we must be open to new evidence all the time.

The experimental method based on the testing of hypotheses has become the orthodoxy of medical science, and this is most clearly demonstrated in the testing of new drugs and treatments. This approach, then, can provide the evidence for medical practice and treatment decisions, provided that the method is ethically and rigorously followed. The RCT appears to be all well and good for providing evidence for some objective truth about the efficacy of pharmaceutical interventions. However, it is not without its critics. Black (1996), for example, has argued that long-term observation studies are needed to evaluate the effectiveness of health care, in addition to RCTs. The established view that the RCT produces the most generalizable evidence is also challenged. Whilst Black accepts that well-designed pharmaceutical trials can be generalized to other settings, he also argues that the uncritical transfer of the RCT to the evaluation of other aspects of health care means that the outcome of trials of surgery, physiotherapy and nursing interventions may be dependent upon the characteristics of the care provider, thus weakening the internal validity of the trial. Whilst Black provides suggestions for overcoming the procedural problems of RCTs, there remain problems of principle, one of which is particularly relevant to the health care of children:

> a randomized trial provides information on the value of an intervention shorn of all context, such as patients' beliefs and wishes and clinicians' attitudes and beliefs, despite the fact that such variables may be crucial to determining the success of the intervention.
>
> (Black, 1996, p. 1218)

This criticism is significant in terms of the discussion which follows for a number of reasons. First, this ethnographic study was concerned with children with asthma. This group of children is of concern to the health professions because of the increase in both the incidence and prevalence of asthma and, despite increasingly sophisticated medication, the fact that children still die from asthma attacks (National Asthma Campaign, 1998). Whilst the RCT can provide evidence for the effectiveness of particular drug regimes, it fails to inform the clinician or parent about the ways in which children interpret their asthma, how they manage it on a daily basis, and how it affects their social identity and interactions with peers, teachers and family. Most importantly, the child's perspective is ignored or overlooked in the classic RCT, and it seems likely that children would be more likely to comply with medical treatment if the regime was constructed around the child's view of him- or herself, rather than the biomedical view. It is in this sense that we propose ethnography can be empowering for children – by providing a different kind of evidence for informing clinical effectiveness, based on the perspective of the child.

Childhood asthma

Asthma is the most common cause of chronic illness in children, particularly those of school age. One study suggests that in the average primary school class of 30 children, four will have asthma (Strachan *et al.*, 1994). The National Asthma Campaign (NAC) audit for 1997/1998 estimates that 1 in 7 children between 2 and 15 years of age have asthma symptoms requiring treatment. The incidence and prevalence of asthma are increasing. The NAC cite Rona *et al.* (1995), whose study of children in England and Scotland revealed an increase in the number of children aged between 5 and 11 years reporting an asthma attack, which was three times higher in 1992 than it was in 1982.

Asthma can vary from a mild condition, requiring a child to use an inhaler for occasional wheeziness, to a serious impediment with frequent episodes of wheezing, coughing and shortness of breath, which may need inhaled medication several times a day. When a child has severe asthma, hospitalization for asthma 'attacks' may be a common occurrence, and if treatment is unsuccessful, asthma can be fatal (Rees, 1989). However, deaths from asthma are falling. In 1995, there were 1621 deaths in total from asthma, which was 44 less than in the previous year (Office of National Statistics, cited by NAC). In view of the high prevalence and rising incidence of childhood asthma, despite an increase in biomedical knowledge of the management of asthma, little research has been conducted on the way in which children, their families and their schools manage asthma on a day-to-day basis (McNabb *et al.*, 1985; Creer *et al.*, 1992).

Concern about the level of patients' and families' understanding and knowledge has grown in the biomedical literature since retrospective studies of families in which a child has died from asthma have shown a substantial lack of information on the part of the patients and parents concerning the disease and its appropriate management (Creer, 1986; Lewiston and Rubinstein, 1987). Ways of sharing biomedical knowledge and skills have been assembled into 'self-management' packages for use by clinicians and health educators with individuals and groups (Creer *et al.*, 1992; Clark *et al.*, 1993; Colland, 1993), with the aim of improving compliance with biomedical regimes of asthma prevention and treatment, so that the condition can be controlled and chronically ill children 'normalised: physically, socially and educationally' (Celano and Geller, 1993). Celano and Geller point out that:

children with asthma may be at risk of school failure due to their symptoms, functional impairments (including school absenteeism) and/or iatrogenic effects of treatment [yet] if their illness is managed effectively, children with asthma can realise their academic potential and enjoy full, productive lives.

(Celano and Geller, 1993)

Armstrong (1983) has argued that the emphasis on normalization results from the increase in biomedical knowledge about children's bodies and the development of child health surveillance during the twentieth century. Children who deviate from the 'norm' are categorized according to their disease or handicap – marked and marginalized as 'others' with respect to 'normal' children. It is this tendency, within the biomedical literature, to emphasize the merits of normalization which we attempted to challenge through our ethnographic study of the way in which children with asthma construct a variety of positive social identities, differing from what might be considered to be 'normal'. We have reported on the construction of social identity elsewhere (Hepper *et al.*, 1996), and therefore the emphasis of this paper is on the potential of this approach to provide an alternative knowledge base to the orthodox, logical empiricist approach to evidence-based health care.

Empowering children?

The very notion of empowering children should probably be challenged at this point. The term makes the assumption that children in general, and specifically children with a chronic disease such as asthma, are powerless both individually and as a social group. Whilst it is true, as has been indicated above, that the perceived powerful medical community has attempted to diminish the identity of the child with a chronic illness, this is not to say that children comply with the identity of the disenfranchised 'sick' role, or see themselves as in need of being normalized. Indeed, as our study appeared to show (Hepper *et al.*, 1996), children with asthma can and do negotiate a social identity for themselves which can cast them in a unique and positive role. However, questions remain about the extent to which children are enabled to make choices about their health or to be involved in the decision-making process. As Kalnins *et al.* point out:

Children's perceptions of health may involve priorities, evaluative processes, ideas of what is possible, and social spheres of relevance different from those of adults. It is therefore essential to understand what is special about children rather than to expect them simply to absorb and accept adult definitions.

(Kalnins *et al.*, 1992, p. 54)

It is in this sense that it may be acceptable to think in terms of empowering children – not as victims of disease, but as powerful individuals who have views and understandings which deserve to be heard. By listening to children it may be possible to construct approaches to health care which match their own priorities and spheres of relevance, whilst at the same time preserving the guiding and protective function of the adult world. Helen Roberts has discussed this in relation to children and policy-making around accident prevention in Chapter 6 of this volume. She presents an analysis of how it might be possible to improve the safety of children by understanding their priorities about risk-taking.

There is a considerable body of research on children's views of health in general – their perceptions of healthy behaviours (e.g. Dielman *et al.*, 1982), what being healthy means to them (e.g. Backett and Alexander, 1991), and how they decide on health actions (Kalnins *et al.*, 1991). Such studies provide an essential flavour of children's perceptions, but it is inappropriate to generalize from these to children who have specific health-related 'problems'. The child with a chronic disease such as asthma may not share the views of a child who has not experienced severe breathlessness, or the look of peers when the inhaler is used, or the need to absent oneself from sports.

Much of the research already cited relied on interviews and conversations to elicit children's perceptions of health. Whilst the interview is one of the most potentially useful research tools, it also presents the researcher with the problem of the relationship between the interviewer (usually an adult) and the interviewee (the child). This in itself creates a potential barrier to the child responding as he or she would really like to, or as he or she thinks the adult would like to hear. Interestingly, Alderson *et al.* (1994) conducted a study in which they trained young people to become interviewers of children in hospital. They found not only that it was possible to train young people to be perceptive and skilled interviewers, but also that their ability to relate to the children they were interviewing led to better quality data than might have been obtained by an adult interviewer. The young people tended to challenge traditional (adult) notions of interviewing, such as talking about oneself, and used their own experiences of hospital to encourage the children to talk.

Observational studies using ethnographic techniques enable the researcher to observe the child in a naturalistic setting and to make careful observations of the day-to-day encounters in which children participate. This can be especially valuable in research on children with a chronic disease, as it enables the researcher to observe a range of interactions over time, rather than the snapshot view that a one-off interview can present. Obviously children in any context vary from day to day, but an interview with a child on a 'wheezy' day might be extremely different to one conducted on a 'good' day. As a participant observer, the researcher was able to note the nuances in the children's behaviour and interactions on a day-to-day basis, as well as listening to what they had to say, when they wanted to say it. She (FH) was quickly absorbed by the children into their everyday lives at school. Children are accustomed to play leaders, teaching assistants, student teachers and young people on work experience (to name but a few) being present in the classroom, playground and sports environment, and in our experience had no apparent difficulty in accepting the researcher into their world, albeit on their terms. Mayall (1994), in her study of children's negotiations of health at school and at home, also used an ethnographic approach. Whilst her study focused, like others, on primary school children in general, Mayall was also concerned with her role in the setting. She found the use of stories, drawings and group discussions enabled children to discuss openly their views on health, as well as making informal observations about their school life and conducting more formal interviews with parents and teachers. Time constraints on our relatively small-scale study precluded the use of interviews with parents. Whilst informal exchanges took place with school staff, the focus was almost exclusively on the observation of children with asthma in their natural social setting. It was the analysis of these observations which led us to consider the extent to which children are constrained in their options in relation to the management of their asthma at school. Constraints (such as limited access to medication) can have the effect of the child being seen as deviant and disruptive by other children and teachers, when the child is in fact trying to construct for him- or herself a 'normal' social identity (see below for an expansion of this discussion). The uncovering of the subtleties of the constraints is what we would describe as potentially empowering for children with asthma. By developing an understanding of the social world of the child with asthma, those in authority can hopefully make simple adjustments to school life which ease their social relationships and facilitate their decision-making. James and Prout (1990), authorities on the anthropology of childhood, have summed up these views as follows:

> Essentially it begins with a construction of the child as an active, participating presence in the social world, rather than a mere passive spectator, and envisages children as having some part in determining the shape which their own lives take. The real promise of the ethnographic approach which it advocates lies in allowing children to have a direct voice and participation in the production of sociological data and for them to be seen as active in the construction and determination of their own social lives, the lives of those around them and the societies in which they live.
>
> (James and Prout, 1990, p. 8)

The ethnography

Context

The fieldwork for this study was conducted in a North London primary school over the autumn term of 1994. The school is comparatively large, with approximately 400 children on its register, although with a mobile population the numbers tend to vary from week to week. The school has a nursery for 3-year-olds, a reception year and six primary years for children aged between 4 and 11 years. The school is situated in the midst of three differing localities and draws children from each of these, resulting in a diversity of ethnic and socio-economic backgrounds. The play areas are divided to meet the needs of different age groups – a soft play area for younger children, and basketball nets and sheds to sit in for the older ones. There is also a football pitch which is fenced off. The school perimeter is screened from the busy main road by trees, but none the less the children are exposed to traffic fumes, especially during the commuter rush-hour, and to fast-moving traffic when crossing the road at home time. The school building is a Victorian construction on several floors, with high ceilings and tall glass windows through which the light floods.

The researcher (FH) was introduced to the school as a local mother, but for the purposes of the research she was accepted by the headteacher, Ms Murray, as a researcher and doctor. The fact that she is a medical doctor (although with no specialist knowledge of asthma) gave the research, in the headteacher's view, legitimacy, and throughout the project she received FH as someone with authority in whom she could confide about the children. This may have distorted the interviews which she freely gave with FH. However, Ms Murray revealed her personal view that asthma was largely psychologically and emotionally mediated. She thereby attributed individual responsibility and personal control to asthma, which became an important theme throughout the ethnography.

The welfare assistants in the school, who were assigned the role of administering the children's medication, were also aware of FH's medical status, which for them raised some anxieties about their own procedures. FH was occasionally in the difficult position of having to give medical advice, whereas her role was to observe and participate in the existing asthma management, rather than to alter practice. This again may have resulted in some distortions in the data, but overall it was acknowledged to be more important that FH revealed her medical status than for her to act covertly, as this would have been professionally unethical and could have raised problems as the fieldwork progressed.

The children primarily accepted FH as a mother of a schoolchild and also, when they realized she was not a teacher, as an adult friend who was interested in finding out about illness at school. Gradually, however, children attending the welfare room where some of the observation took place came to understand that FH was also a doctor. For some, this helped them to explain why she was interested in their views on being ill at school.

The school policy for the management of illness and medication at school covered the management of asthma. It decreed that parents should supply the required medication with written instructions, and that welfare assistants should comply with these instructions, the medication being kept by the welfare assistant in the welfare room. A tight set of guidelines to ensure continuous surveillance of the children governed their need to be excused from class time to take medication. For example, a child would be required to carry a card indicating permission to be absent from class to attend the welfare room. Emergency situations were well catered for within the policy, although the guidelines might have been interpreted as somewhat rigid in the event of a serious emergency. The overall tone of the policy was one of maintaining discipline and non-disruptive behaviour in the face of illness requiring regular medication, as was the case for many of the children with asthma.

The majority of the fieldwork took place in the classrooms of years five and six. This involved 90 children in total, of whom 15 individuals were 'officially' described as having asthma, which is a little higher than the figure of 1 in 7 discussed in the literature (National Asthma Campaign, 1998). The researcher became aware of a few children who were not on the official list because their parents had not written to the school about the asthma and/or the children had not handed over their medication. Because of the known pressures of the national curriculum, much of the observation took place quietly and discreetly, and children were encouraged to talk to FH during playtime and in preparation for sports (for example, on the coach which took them to swimming lessons), rather than in class. The classroom observation led to much insight into how the children negotiate their asthma in a rigidly surveyed, individualized setting, and how these negotiations compared with others in different settings in the school.

Children's negotiations of 'having asthma'

This section will focus on that part of the ethnography which led to our interpretations of the way in which children negotiate their way through what Comaroff (1981) has described as a disordering event that implies deviation from a common universe of experience and a disruption of existing personal relationships, activities and social roles.

One of the themes that emerged from talking to the staff, noting the various school policies and observing the way in which the children behaved and were expected to behave was the emphasis placed by the school on individualism and responsibility for self. This was driven by the head-teacher, who in her own observations of some of the children with asthma described those children whose asthma was well managed as 'good boys who rarely give us any trouble', and other children such as Ayesha as 'over-anxious', implying that she was not in control of her emotions, and Hamed as 'over-determined' and disruptive. Asthma was seen to be a disruption of school life which, like other types of disruption, should be under individual control. Disruption of any kind in the classroom could therefore be punished by exclusion – for bad behaviour children were sent to Ms Murray, and for wheeziness they were sent to the welfare room or had to miss sports. Sometimes children would describe how they would try to cope with wheezing rather than be seen to disrupt the class and go through the lengthy surveillance system to acquire their inhaler and therefore identify themselves as 'different'. However, through the lens of the ethnographer it became apparent that these children were challenging the notion that to be a person one must be 'in control' in a uniform manner. The children's experience was frequently one of not being in control, in the sense of controlling themselves to be like everybody else, within the boundaries of a uniform 'normality'. Instead they constituted ways of being 'differently normal' which did not threaten them. The means by which children with asthma negotiated this 'different normality' can be classified into means of resistance, accommodation and transformation, illustrated by the following case examples.

Resistance

Children found ways of resisting the interest of others in the differences signified by their asthma, rendering them less conspicuous. Hamed was an expert at this approach. He would frequently return to the classroom late after playtime, returning from the welfare room after using his inhaler to relieve wheeziness after an energetic football match. (This was perceived by the class teacher to be disruptive and inappropriate behaviour, but was important to Hamed to maintain his identity as a footballer.) On one occasion he sidled into the classroom 10 minutes late. When the boy next to him started to ask questions about his whereabouts, Hamed turned away with his book and shielded himself from the other boy's surveillance with his arm. When the questions persisted, Hamed simply removed himself from the situation by moving over to the library and working at a different table.

Accommodation

In one of the year groups at the school there were eight girls with asthma, six of whom were closely bonded in a friendship group which included another girl, Emma, who did not have asthma.

The girls liked to meet with FH and talk about their experiences of asthma. During the course of their discussions, FH came to appreciate the significance of the shared experience of having asthma and how it was accommodated into a sense of what they shared about each other. Emma 'looked after' them all and always sat at the side of the playground with whoever was too wheezy to play. The group frequented each other's homes, feeling safe because they 'knew what to do' in the event of an asthma attack. Rather than being a threat to them, the lack of 'self-control' experienced by these girls with asthma actually strengthened their sense of belonging to one another and being able to care for one another. Their own sense of control came from taking turns at being dependent and dependable. As Murphy (1987) has argued with regard to disability, whilst dependency is a problem which all disabled people face, reliance on another person can be encompassed by love and feelings of mutuality.

Transformation

On one occasion, Mandy, in year six, began a terrible and prolonged coughing fit in class. She tried to shield herself from the stares of the other children by burying her head in her arms, but eventually the teacher had to stop talking, as she could no longer be heard. Other children began to laugh, and it took a few minutes for the teacher to bring this disruption to the class under control. The teacher turned to Mandy and asked her if she thought she should go swimming. Mandy said she thought she should, and that she had her inhaler. The teacher felt that this cough required more than an inhaler: 'it's a chesty cough – you need medicine, if you go swimming it takes up . . . you need a lot of air'. A further bout of coughing brought Mandy to the attention of the class again – smiles and sniggers ensued. The teacher's response was to admonish the class for bad behaviour and to say to Mandy 'I really don't think you should go swimming . . . but I can't decide for you, it's your responsibility'.

Whilst the above incident appears to describe the teacher's judgement that Mandy's cough is a possible cause of exclusion from swimming, the children's response to Mandy's cough is similar to that of other disruptions caused by 'mucking about' in class – a kind of embarrassed amusement at Mandy's flaunting of authority. During the course of this episode, the disruption of asthma was transformed, through the interaction of the class, into disruption due to 'mucking about'. Mandy became the subject of appraisal in the children's eyes through her apparent flaunting of authority. The transfer of focus from her symptoms to her behaviour averted the threat to Mandy as a person lacking in 'self-control'. Rather, she was placed in a position of control by the teacher and asked whether she should go swimming or not. Of course it is difficult to judge the extent to which individual children manipulate the possibilities for transformation to occur, but as a strategy for avoiding exclusion and turning perceived lack of control into appraisal, it was very effective.

These three examples show how children whose bodies had been rendered different by asthma engaged in situations and experiences which challenged the explicit messages that were being delivered through the moral curriculum of individual responsibility which made 'self-control' and 'self-discipline' such essential attributes of what it is to be a person. Often not 'in control', they none the less found ways of being integrated as valued individuals in their social world.

Conclusions

This chapter has drawn on the observation of children with asthma in one school in an attempt to show how children negotiate and construct their own identities as people with a chronic disease. In the process, we have also attempted to show that ethnography can result in a different kind of evidence to inform policy and practice through the revealing of the management of asthma from a child's perspective. Rather than a child being necessarily identified as different or deviant by himself or peers, we have shown through case examples how children re-negotiate themselves as 'differently normal' through either resistance, accommodation or transformation. We argued earlier in this chapter that ethnography may in itself be empowering for children with asthma (or any chronic condition). It remains difficult for us to envisage how the insights which were gained from this study of children's management of asthma at school could have been obtained through other methods which use a more positivist approach. In this sense, the children in this study may have been empowered to inform the world of health and biomedicine about the way in which they construct their own approach to asthma. We had envisaged examples of stigmatization and social exclusion of children by their peers, but found instead that children with asthma were often accommodated into the social group and well able to manage their asthma in a way which did not stigmatize them. The aims of many biomedically determined self-management programmes may therefore not be so relevant if children sustain self and social identities of different normality. Rather than focusing on problems of non-compliance with treatment and difficulties of being absent from school or sports and other activities, it may be more appropriate to focus attention on the ways in which children successfully negotiate their identities, and to base education about asthma and other disabilities on positive notions of becoming a person. Such interventions have been described by Kalnins *et al.* (1992) and others as Lifeskills programmes. Tones touches on this approach to health education in Chapter 3. The challenge is to institute such programmes for children with chronic diseases into schools and to conduct proper evaluations of their worth, by which we would include children's views as well as outcomes. For example, working with mixed groups of children and using case examples and their own experiences may help to engender positive attitudes towards disability, as well as providing strategies for children to explore.

Clearly, from a positivist perspective we could be accused of making broad generalizations based on a small-scale study. Certainly it is not being asserted that, on the basis of this study, all children with asthma respond in this way. A longer and more detailed observation study would enable us to confirm and strengthen the theories presented here. Nor is it proposed that all educational programmes for children with asthma should be dismantled on the basis of this study – these will always provide a sound knowledge base and a rationale for treating the symptoms of asthma. Our contention is that there is evidence from this study which contests biomedical orthodoxy in relation to the management of asthma at school, and that this should be taken into account when designing new programmes in school health and setting policy in schools for asthma management. For example, at the outset of this study we considered that it would be more empowering for children if they were allowed to carry their own inhalers, and not subjected to the potentially differentiating and socially isolating experience of having to excuse themselves from class to relieve asthma symptoms. However, our interpretation of the ethnography would lead us to question whether, by introducing a policy where children have complete control over their medication they in fact, through forced publicity, have less control over their identity and are seen as disruptive or deviant. Whilst it is possible that familiarity through the everyday use of inhalers might render the experience of having asthma an ordinary part of school life, it is equally possible that the spectacle of asthma would signify children as extraordinary and make it more difficult for them to be accommodated. In Geertz's (1983) terms, the experiences of children in this study challenged adult notions of an egocentric concept of personhood and constituted instead a socio-centric formulation, where a person's worth is conceived of in terms of his or her relationship to others. Children's negotiations in this respect might change to a more egocentric sense of self if further self-controlling and self-surveillance mechanisms were placed upon them through the management of their own medication. Further study of an environment in which children do carry their own medication would add further validity to these claims and help to answer questions about children having more control over their disability. Finally, Stallibrass (1989) has noted that 'the ability to exercise choice and to learn by doing are crucial elements in the environment and that adult "experts" may be obstacles to children's realisation of what is important and satisfying'. The study described here supports this view, but has also helped to uncover some of the ways in which children with a debilitating condition can successfully negotiate their own way through the adult world.

References

Alderson, P. 1994: *Listening to children – children, ethics and social research.* London: Barnardo's.

Armstrong, D. 1983: *Political anatomy of the body: medical knowledge in Britain in the twentieth century.* Cambridge: Cambridge University Press.

Backett, K. and Alexander, H. 1991: Talking to young children about health: methods and findings. *Health Education Journal* **50**, 34–8.

Black, N. 1996: Why we need observational studies to evaluate the effectiveness of health care. *British Medical Journal* **312**, 1215–18.

Carr, W. and Kemmis, S. 1986: *Becoming critical. Education, knowledge and action research.* London: Falmer Press.

Celano, M. and Geller, R. 1993: Learning, school performance and children with asthma: how much at risk? *Journal of Learning Disabilities* **26**, 23–32.

Clark, N.M., Gotch, A. and Rosenstock, I.R. 1993: Patient, professional and public education on behavioural aspects of asthma: a review of strategies for change and need research. *Journal of Asthma* **30**, 241–55.

Colland, V. 1993: Learning to cope with asthma: a behavioural self-management program for children. *Patient Education and Counselling* **22**, 141–52.

Comaroff, J. 1981: Healing and cultural transformation: the Tswana of Southern Africa. *Social Science and Medicine* **15B**, 367–78.

Creer, T. 1986: Psychological factors and death from asthma: creation and critique of a myth. *Journal of Asthma* **23**, 261–9.

Creer, T.L., Stein, R.E., Rappaport, L. and Lewis, C. 1992: Behavioural consequences of illness: childhood asthma as a model. *Paediatrics* **90**, 808–15.

Dielman, T., Leech, S., Becker, M., Rosenstock, I., Horvath, W. and Radius, S. 1982: Parental and child health beliefs and behaviour. *Health Education Quarterly* **9**, 56–60.

Geertz, C. 1983: From the native's point of view: on the nature of anthropological understanding. In Geertz, C. (ed.), *Local knowledge*. New York: Basic Books.

Hammersley, M. and Atkinson, P. 1995: *Ethnography – principles in practice*, 2nd edn. London: Routledge.

Hepper, F., Robinson, I. and Kendall, S. 1996: Significantly different or successfully unique?: an asthmatic child's construction of social identity. *British Medical Anthropology Review* **3**, 5–10.

James, A. and Prout, A. 1990: A new paradigm for the sociology of childhood? Provenance, promise or problem? In James, A. and Prout, A. (eds), *Constructing and reconstructing childhood; contemporary issues in the sociological study of childhood*. Basingstoke: Falmer Press, 7–34.

Kalnins, I., Yoshida, M. and Kellmer, M. 1991: Decision-making strategies of 9–12 year old children in everyday situations involving their health. Unpublished paper.

Kalnins, I., McQueen, D., Backett, K., Curtice, L. and Currie, C. 1992: Children, empowerment and health promotion: some new directions in research and practice. *Health Promotion International* **7**, 53–9.

Kleinman, A., Eisenberg, L. and Good, B. 1978: Culture, illness and care. *Annals of Internal Medicine* **88**, 251–8.

Lather, P. 1994: Critical inquiry in qualitative research. Feminist and post-structural perspectives: science 'after truth'. In Crabtree, B.F., Miller, W.L., Addison, R.B., Gilchrist, V.J. and Kigel, A.J. (eds), *Exploring collaborative research in primary care*. London: Sage, 103–14.

Lewiston, N.J. and Rubinstein, S. 1987: The young Damocles: the adolescent at high risk for serious or fatal status asthmaticus. *Clinical Review of Allergy* **5**, 273–84.

Lincoln, Y. and Guba, E. 1985: *Naturalistic inquiry*. Beverly Hills, CA: Sage.

McNabb, W.L., Wilson-Pessano, S.R. and Jacobs, A.M. 1985: Critical self-management competencies for children with asthma. *Journal of Paediatric Psychology* **11**, 101–17.

Mayall, B. 1994: *Negotiating health – primary school children at home and school*. London: Cassell.

Murphy, R. 1987: *The body silent*. London: Phoenix House.

National Asthma Campaign 1998: *National Asthma Audit 1997/98*. London: National Asthma Campaign.

National Health Service Executive 1996: *Primary care led NHS: briefing pack*. London: National Health Service Executive.

Popper, K. 1959: *The logic of scientific discovery*. London: Hutchinson.

Rees, J. 1989: *ABC of Asthma*. London: BMJ Publications.

Rona, R., Chinn, S. and Burney, P. 1995: Trends in the prevalence of asthma in Scottish and English primary school children 1982–1992. *Thorax* **50**, 992–3.

Sackett, D., Rosenberg, W., Muir Gray, J.A., Haynes, R.B. and Richardson, W.S. 1996: Evidence-based medicine: what it is and what it isn't. *British Medical Journal* **312**, 71–2.

Stallibrass, A. 1989: *Being me and also us: lessons from the Peckham experiment.* Edinburgh: Scottish Academic Press.

Strachan, D., Anderson, H., Limb, E., O'Neill, A. and Wells, N. 1994: A national survey of asthma prevalence, severity and treatment in Great Britain. *Archives of Disease in Childhood* **70**, 174–8.

8

Empowerment and breastfeeding

Margaret Gordon

Introduction

In most European countries the incidence of breastfeeding has declined spectacularly during the present century. The tendency to bottle-feed has gained momentum in most western countries over this period, mainly because of the lead taken by the USA. The decline in breastfeeding has been attributed to a wide range of factors, including the following: the increase in the number of women working outside the home; the majority of babies being delivered in a hospital setting where healthy mothers are described as 'patients'; medical supervision and, in fact, regimentation of infant feeding in the postpartum period; adoption of a technical approach to the management of lactation; high-profile marketing of formula milk; and the failure of most health professionals to give support and encouragement for breastfeeding (Brunn, 1986; Kassianos, 1993).

The incidence of breastfeeding in Northern Ireland must be ranked as one of the lowest in Europe, and as a nation it could be described as a 'bottle-feeding' culture. A multiplicity of factors impinge on the incidence and duration of breastfeeding, and therefore it is not merely a matter of having the correct information. Complex cultural conditioning and relationships come into play. It has been shown that factors such as race, religion, culture and gender may influence health knowledge, attitudes and behaviour (Calnan, 1986; Backett, 1992; Kendall, 1995).

Breastfeeding as an art rather than an instinct is a behaviour optimized by experience, observation of role models, and information and support from health professionals and society in general. As fewer and fewer mothers attempt the art of breastfeeding in Northern Ireland, the decreasing trend continues to result in fewer mothers and babies reaping the known health gains associated with the practice. The nutritional and developmental values of breastfeeding are well documented in the literature, and the body of scientific knowledge in its favour continues to grow.

Whilst many factors have been cited as contributing to the successes and failures of breastfeeding, it is apparent that many women frequently express disappointment in the support offered to them by the health professionals who, in theory, should be suitably informed and strategically placed to facilitate their infant-feeding choice and to support them in their efforts. Moreover, the 'pool' of knowledge and skills among mothers has decreased. The way in which parents are cared for during pregnancy and childbirth is crucial for laying the foundations of confidence and self-esteem. Care that empowers women involves respect, acknowledgment of their concerns, information-giving and the offering of choice (Niven, 1992). A new model of professional practice is emerging, one in which professionals see themselves as empowering rather than controlling, working in partnership with service users to help them to gain control over their own world rather than conform to that of professionals. Such professionals recognize and respect service users' experience, knowledge and skills, and make their own professional knowledge and expertise available to users. They do not impose their own priorities and perspectives, nor do they seek to take responsibility from users in order to fulfil their own needs. Their base of power rests in personal security, not professional status, and their claim to professionalism rests on their ability to facilitate and enable, not to direct and control. Fahlberg *et al.* (1991) suggest that the route to this new form of 'empowering' professional practice is through the empowerment of professionals themselves.

The following chapter gives an account of some recent initiatives carried out in Northern Ireland in an attempt to nurture the country back to being a breastfeeding nation. It will commence with a review of the most recent evidence relating breastfeeding to health gains for both mothers and babies, and will then go on to examine some of the obstacles placed in the way of breastfeeding in Northern Ireland, describe local training initiatives aimed at empowering health professionals, and how these impacted on practice, and the resultant effects on the incidence of breastfeeding locally.

The case for promoting breastfeeding in Northern Ireland: the health gains

Protection against infection

Many health gains for the mother and baby have been illuminated in relation to breastfeeding. These are not only beneficial to society at large, but must also be of interest to the managers of an efficient and effective health service – because breastfeeding not only maximizes health but is also cost-effective. Researchers in the USA have identified the high national costs as a result of the iatrogenic ill health that results from bottle-feeding (Facione, 1990;

Walker, 1993). Palmer (1993a) has reported that in the UK, regardless of socio-economic conditions, a bottle-fed baby is five times more likely to suffer from gastrointestinal illness in the first 3 months of life than a breastfed baby. It costs around £300 per day to care for a baby in hospital. In 1991 it cost one English town £225 000 to hospitalize 150 such babies for 3–7 days each. At that rate, if 300 UK towns achieved the breastfeeding rates of Norway (90 per cent at 3 months) or Finland (95 per cent initiation, 75–86 per cent at 6 months) (World Health Organization, 1990), the National Health Service would save over £67 million a year (Palmer, 1993b).

Studies that have compared artificial feeding with breastfeeding generally agreed that breastfeeding protects babies from gastrointestinal infections. In a review of over 40 studies since 1970, Baucher *et al.* (1986) concluded that breastfeeding had a protective effect in industrial countries, despite the fact that some methodology was, in his opinion, flawed. Cunningham (1987) vigorously disputed the latter, as did Howie and Forsyth (1990) in a Dundee study of 618 children, who found that babies who were breastfed for 13 weeks not only had protection, but the benefits lasted up to 1 year of age. There was thus a higher incidence of hospital admissions among formula-fed babies. Baucher *et al.* (1986) assessed the extent to which studies of the association between breastfeeding and infections met four methodological standards that relate to both scientific validity and generalizability of the studies. The four methodological studies that were applicable to these studies were adopted from the work of Horwitz and Feinstein (1979) and Feinstein (1985). These were avoidance of detection bias, adjustments for potential confounding variables, definition of the outcome event, and a clear definition of what was meant by 'breastfeeding'. The study carried out in Dundee by Howie *et al.* (1990) was the first large UK study with more than 500 subjects. This study design was in keeping with recommendations by Baucher *et al.* (1986), as 500 subjects was the minimum sample size to have sufficient power to investigate the relationship fully. It showed clearly that breastfed babies were healthier and less likely to suffer from respiratory infections and gastroenteritis.

The effects of breastfeeding on respiratory illness have been studied in Wales by Burr (1989), who concluded that any breastfeeding appeared to halve the risk of wheezing in infants followed up to 1 year. It has also been shown to be prophylactic against atopic disease, with the effect extending into adulthood. Breastfeeding for longer than 1 month without other milk supplements offers significant prophylaxis against food allergy at 3 years of age, and also against respiratory allergy at 17 years of age. Six months of breastfeeding are required to prevent eczema during the first 3 years, and possibly also to prevent substantial atropy in adolescence (Saarinen and Kajoasaari, 1995). These results were similar to those found earlier in a 20-year UK follow-up study (Blair, 1977).

Pisacane (1994), in Italian studies, also suggested that breastfeeding had a strong protective effect against acute lower respiratory infection. Pisacane

(1990) also found that breast milk protected babies from urinary tract infection (UTI). UTI can have a lasting detrimental effect on children, and costs millions of pounds a year in health care treatment.

Breastfeeding has been shown to reduce the development of otitis media during the first year of life (Duncan and Holberg, 1993). It was found that babies who were exclusively breastfed had half the number of episodes of otitis media compared to those who received no breast milk at all. The incidence of children attending GP clinics with ear infection is always on the increase. Prophylaxis in the form of breastfeeding may protect children from repeated doses of antibiotic therapy.

Mortality

It is difficult to assess the mortality of breastfed compared to formula-fed infants at present, because many breastfed infants also received supplements of formula and solid foods. The risk of death in the first year of life has diminished in developed countries during this century, since the advent of antibiotics and many other advances in paediatric care (Sloper *et al.*, 1974). However, data from other nations do show a significant difference (Grulee *et al.*, 1986).

UNICEF regularly states in the literature that over a million babies die from unsafe bottle-feeding every year, and it estimates that babies who are bottle-fed in poor countries are 25 times more likely to die than breastfed babies.

With regard to the topical subject of sudden infant death syndrome (SIDS), Savage (1992) quoted evidence from the Avon infant mortality study and the New Zealand cot death study, suggesting important risk factors for SIDS (Mitchell *et al.*, 1991). Whilst sleeping position, cot mattress and parental smoking attracted media attention, breastfeeding failed to reach the headlines despite the significance of the following risk factors for SIDS:

- sleeping prone – 5.74
- tobacco use – 1.83
- *not* breastfed – 2.45

The importance of breastfeeding as a risk-lowering factor has also been shown by other investigators (Dumas *et al.*, 1988).

This clearly indicates a significant risk reduction when a child is breastfed. The benefits of breastfeeding should be taught to all mothers in order to reduce the risk.

Breastfeeding and intellectual development

The burden of proof has always lain with breast milk, yet new research continually evidences its superiority. Long-chain fatty acids and neurological advantage are but one of the most recent topics to emerge. Breastfeeding is better for babies' brains, as has been shown in a recent study at Glasgow's Royal Hospital for Sick Children. Significantly more docosahexaenoic acid (DHA) was found in the cerebral cortex phospholipids of breastfed babies than in those of babies fed on either of two infant formulas (Farquharson, 1995).

Breast milk contains the essential long-chain polyunsaturated fatty acids (LCP), arachidonic acid (AA) and docosahexaenoic acid (DHA). The importance of LCP in breast milk is for brain development, visual development, and for growth of tissue. The brain is composed of 60 per cent lipid, which universally uses arachidonic acid and docosahexaenoic acid for growth, function and integrity. Both acids are consistent components of human milk (Crawford, 1993).

The idea that breastfed babies will be more intelligent is not new. Several studies have reported that children who have been breastfed as babies did better on IQ tests (Morley and Cole, 1988; Lucas *et al.*, 1992). Even after bias towards higher education and socio-economic status have been taken into account, some measurable advantage may remain. Lanting (1994), in studies on 9-year-old children in The Netherlands, suggested that the method of feeding during early childhood also had a long-term effect on cognitive development in both full-term and pre-term infants.

The European Commission has proposed amendments to the Directive on Infant Formulae to require the addition of essential fatty acids, linoleic acid and alpha-linolenic acid within specific limits, but it does not overcome the limited capacity to synthesize longer-chain derivatives (Department of Health, 1994).

Long-term differences in health

The protective benefits of breastfeeding may extend long beyond childhood. Breastfeeding has been associated with lower incidences of coeliac disease (Greco *et al.*, 1988) and Crohn's disease (Kalezko *et al.*, 1989). Both conditions can be debilitating, and may result in periods out of work, with high costs both to the individual and to society at large.

Insulin-dependent diabetics are more likely to have been bottle-fed (Metcalf and Baum, 1992). A case-control investigation of perinatal risk factors for childhood insulin-dependent diabetics in Northern Ireland and Scotland showed a reduction in risk (albeit a small one) among breastfed children (Patterson, 1994). A recent study has even indicated that children with acute appendicitis were less likely to have been breastfed (Pisacane, 1995), as breastfeeding can modify the exposure and/or type of immune response to some microbial agents during infancy. The immune components of human milk provide an antigen avoidance system that can decrease the severity of infection, and probably also the inflammatory reactions associated with it (Goldman, 1993). The milder inflammatory response could programme the immune system of the infant, its effects lasting for several years, and it could be associated with a more tolerant lymphoid tissue at the base of the appendix. Pisacane *et al.* (1996) also found that breastfed children were less likely to require tonsillectomy.

Contraindications to breastfeeding

The body of evidence continues to grow, demonstrating that despite the health benefits now well known to most if not all mothers, many mothers within Northern Ireland still choose the formula-milk option. It is obvious that many other factors must therefore impinge on a mother's feeding choice or her ability to breastfeed successfully.

American paediatricians suggest that 95 per cent of all women are physiologically capable of breastfeeding (American Academy of Paediatrics, 1982). However, it is also necessary to state that there are occasions when breastfeeding should not be promoted. These include the cases of mothers with the AIDS virus, or mothers who are known drug abusers, in order to avoid the risk of causing infant drug dependency (Soni, 1988). Mothers being treated for medical reasons with certain drugs which may be transmitted through their breast milk (i.e. tetracyclines, lobibes) should not be encouraged to breastfeed. The presence of lactose imbalance, galactosaemia and phenylketonuria are also other known contraindications to breast-feeding (Soni, 1988).

Focusing in particular on the AIDS virus, it has been documented that there have been a small number of cases in which breastfeeding appears to be the significant determining factor in the transmission of HIV from mother to infant. HIV has been cultured from cell-free extracts of breast milk (Thiry, 1985). The presence of HIV-infected cells has also been detected in breast milk. The actual risk of transmission of HIV through breast milk is unknown. One estimate puts the risk of transmission at 29 per cent, based on four studies of mothers who acquired HIV postnatally (Mok, 1993). Analysis of another five studies showed that when the mother was infected antenatally, the additional risk of transmission through breastfeeding, over and above transmission *in utero* or during delivery, was 14 per cent. Breastfeeding is not recommended at present for mothers with HIV in Northern Ireland.

The circumstances listed above are indeed rare and have a minimal effect on the overall incidence of breastfeeding within the province. However, this information had to be included to ensure that the evidence provided was not construed as a universal promotion of breastfeeding.

Promoting breastfeeding in Northern Ireland: the barriers

A survey conducted by the Office of Population Censuses and Surveys for the first time in Northern Ireland in 1990 revealed an incidence of 36 per cent compared to 63 per cent in the UK (White *et al.*, 1992). This figure falls to 25 per cent in County Antrim, one of the lowest rates in Europe. Northern Ireland mothers who do initiate breastfeeding do so for a shorter time than those in England, Scotland and Wales. By 6 weeks after birth, less than half (49 per cent) of Northern Ireland mothers who had initiated breastfeeding were still continuing to do so (White *et al.*, 1992). Culturally, Northern Ireland is now recognized as a bottle-feeding nation.

Whilst many factors influence the infant-feeding choice, the most common reason for terminating breastfeeding early is a perceived lack of milk supply (White *et al.*, 1992). In western society, mothers and grandmothers tend to become obsessed with the fact that the baby is not getting enough milk – sadly this is often reinforced by over-zealous health professionals who frequently weigh and re-weigh infants, focusing only on weight gain, with the unintended consequence of undermining the mother's confidence in her body's natural ability to nourish her child. The introduction of complementary bottles of formula milk also reduces stimulation and/or suckling at the breast, and ultimately reduces milk production. Researchers in Ireland (Murray and Webster, 1988; Becker, 1992) reported similar findings in that they found older, more experienced midwives were less supportive of breastfeeding, and more likely to recommend complementary formula feeds.

Many mothers also claim that, had they received more consistent advice and support from informed health professionals, they might have breastfed for longer and more successfully (Knaft, 1974; Morgan, 1985; Jones, 1986; Rajan, 1993). Sadly, therefore, the evidence for the lack of professional effectiveness has been shown to be one of the first barriers to successful breastfeeding (Countryman, 1973; Cole, 1977). Conflicting advice, lack of support, and professional attitudes that are non-conducive to breastfeeding have all been identified (McKnight, 1987; Murray and Webster, 1988). To compound this, hospital practices have also been shown to hinder breastfeeding. In 1990, 45 per cent of breastfed babies had already received bottle feeds while in hospital, and sadly a clear relationship has been shown between giving bottles of infant formula in hospital and giving up breastfeeding in the first 2 weeks (White *et al.*, 1992). The historical medicalization of childbirth and control of infant nutrition has left us with rigid hospital routines and practices. Voluntary support groups such as the National Childbirth Trust and La Leche have brought to light the neglect of breastfeeding in hospitals, the misleading advice which the doctors and consultants have been giving to women, and the extent to which medical establishments have become compromised by the enormous commercial interests involved in the production and sale of baby formula feeds. Palmer (1993a) stated that medical traditions which destroy breastfeeding were sanctified by recommendations in text books and training schools, and were perpetuated by health professionals.

However, some more positive changes since 1990 have taken place in an attempt to put women at the centre of their own care as recommended in the

Winterton Report (House of Commons Select Committee on Health, 1992) – the first report of its kind to include evidence from women themselves. This idea was reaffirmed, and more clearly defined, in *Changing Childbirth* (Department of Health, 1993). In order to nurture a child, a woman needs to feel valued and nurtured herself (Kitzinger, 1983). She needs to have confidence in her own ability to think clearly and to make good decisions for herself and her baby. This clearly makes new demands on health professionals, who all too often in the past have been known for their paternalism. A further positive influencing factor has come from the Baby-Friendly Hospital Initiative – a global programme run jointly by the World Health Organization (WHO) and the United Nations Children's Fund (UNICEF) – which aims to promote improved support by maternity hospital staff to mothers who wish to breastfeed. Maternity hospitals are invited to apply for accreditation, which involves an external inspection team evaluating hospital practice in relation to each of the 10 WHO-UNICEF standards of practice. However, according to the current regulations, a hospital must achieve a hospital breastfeeding rate of at least 75 per cent to be able to qualify for Baby-Friendly Hospital accreditation. Whilst no hospital in Northern Ireland could at present attain a 75 per cent incidence of breastfeeding, several are in fact currently striving to qualify for at least some of the Baby-Friendly Hospital stages – when the Baby-Friendly Initiative was launched in Northern Ireland in 1995, a staged method of accreditation was offered across the province.

In Northern Ireland, however, mothers still have to deal with the considerable muddles in obstetric and paediatric practice and tradition derived from the fact that the medical professional envisages mothers and babies as belonging to different fields of research. When a mother and baby are separated so that the baby can be treated in a special-care baby unit, infant nutrition is then considered under the domain of the paediatrician, whilst maternal care rests with the gynaecologist – this is surely an unnatural division of care particularly when the mother desires to breastfeed. The breastfeeding dyad is therefore separated in order to accommodate different medical specialists.

Whilst many changes have occurred in Northern Ireland within the hospital setting, much still needs to be achieved. Unrestricted contact between mother and baby following delivery, demand feeding, and rooming in are now all evidenced in most large maternity units within the province. However, no maternity unit in Northern Ireland would claim to have achieved all of the '10 steps to successful breastfeeding' – the global criteria required by UNICEF to designate a hospital as 'Baby Friendly'. The Office of Population Censuses and Surveys (White *et al.*, 1992) provides some evidence that practices in maternity units do not always conform to recommendations for good care. For example, it found that nearly half of the breastfed babies had been given bottles of artificial milk in the first week, and this proportion has changed little since the 1980s. Postnatal wards are often full of mothers lying gazing at their babies through the sides of cots or reaching out to touch them, when often what they really want is to be with and maintain skin contact with their young. Taking babies into bed in Northern Ireland in some areas would still be frowned upon – daring to fall asleep with them may well result in a reprimand.

Moss (1990), in her qualitative research study – based in County Antrim – called 'breastfeeding in a bottle-feeding world', found that there were often insufficient experienced staff with the time (and possibly the motivation) to help and support the nursing mother. In Londonderry, Murray and Webster (1988) noted that one of the factors contributing to low rates of breastfeeding was a lack of enthusiasm for promoting breastfeeding reported by the midwives, which in turn related to their lack of appreciation of the value of breastfeeding. McKnight (1987), in a Belfast study, also stated that many health professionals now seem to favour the view that bottle-feeding is just as good as breastfeeding, and do not therefore give encouragement or restore confidence when that is all that is often required. Relative lack of support and encouragement identified both in hospital and in the community may be partly a product of staff attitudes. This is rather damning for accountable health professionals, yet in the context of a society where so few choose to breastfeed, including many of these health professionals themselves, can they be held totally culpable? As a decreasing number of mothers in Northern Ireland breastfeed, fewer health professionals seem to have the skills to support mothers through a normal successful breastfeeding experience. Problems arise more often than they should. Health professionals, it would appear, often lack the skills to help mothers and fathers to overcome problems, and breastfeeding fails more often than it should. It is clear that nurses have failed to provide specific information about – and support for – breastfeeding (Knaft, 1974; Jones, 1986). Several authors (Countryman, 1973; Cole, 1977; Whitley, 1978) indicate that nurses often lack the requisite knowledge to assist women adequately to breastfeed. In our society, as fewer mothers choose to breastfeed, there are fewer role models, and most definitely little or no breastfeeding viewed in public. In Northern Ireland it is often socially unacceptable to be seen breastfeeding in public places (Moss, 1990). Many nurses would also claim that their traditional training ill equips them for the task. Cultural information about breastfeeding has almost disappeared, so mothers often turn to health professionals for help, and sadly it appears that they are often poorly equipped to help. Since research evidence has shown that the reasons for stopping breastfeeding are often linked with the educational approach adopted by health professionals, clearly there was a need to reassess the obstacles placed in the way of breastfeeding by inappropriate practices and advice. However, more important still, there was a need to re-acquire the skills needed to help mothers to breastfeed successfully. It must be noted that it was not only professional knowledge levels, but also their attitudes and practice that influence the information and quality of support offered to mothers and fathers.

The 'lost art' of breastfeeding appears to be one of the reasons for the failure of women to continue breastfeeding. As Palmer says, breastfeeding is not an instinct any more, and is something which now has to be learned (Palmer, 1993a). Health professionals therefore need to be knowledgeable and skilled in order to support a mother through a normal breastfeeding experience. It is well known that extra interest in, and support for, breastfeeding can increase its success (Burne, 1976). Michin states:

> The discrepancy between those women who are capable of breastfeeding and those who succeed may pin-point weaknesses among those who support them rather than the women themselves. Indeed, one Australian writer attributes a large part of the responsibility for breastfeeding failure to professional ignorance. She continues: I am not imputing negligence or stupidity or malice, or making any other moral judgements. I know that most professionals are hard-working, humane, and dedicated. I am reporting that there is a degree of professional ignorance which is historically quite understandable, but no longer tolerable.
>
> (Michin, 1985, p. xi)

It has been assumed that it is the health professionals, in particular midwives and health visitors, who are the key people responsible for making breastfeeding happen. Their challenge is not just to acquire skills and knowledge, but also to function in an environment where a rich baby-food industry gives very clear messages about the benefits of their products, and where the World Health Organization/UNICEF code (World Health Organization, 1987) of marketing of breast milk substitutes has not been recognized as serious legislation. Training to empower health professionals to promote and maintain breastfeeding in the 'real world' is essential.

Empowering health professionals and mothers to breastfeed in Northern Ireland

If the health professionals in Northern Ireland are to empower Northern Ireland mothers to breastfeed, they themselves must first be empowered. In a broad sense, empowerment is a process by which people, organizations and communities gain mastery over their own lives, and implies that many competencies are present, or possible, given the right opportunities (Rappaport, 1984). Kalnins (1992) stated that empowered people must feel that they have significant control over their health and the conditions that affect their health. The individual woman will be empowered when she is able to communicate her wishes effectively, when others involved in her care communicate fully with her, when she has a say in decisions which affect her and her baby, when she has sufficient knowledge to make decisions and choices, when she has real choice, and when she is treated with respect and supported in the choices she has made (Shelton, 1994). Empowerment depends on informed choice. Both information and choices are essential to a woman's decisions about the care of her children. Wallerstein and Bernstein (1988) state that empowerment involves much more than increasing one's self-esteem and self-efficacy, or promoting positive health behaviour in individuals. It involves environmental change too. Butterfield (1990) notes the need to understand the complex social, political and economic forces that shape people's lives. Breastfeeding is not merely a nutritional matter, with mothers as people needing to be informed of its importance. Interventions cannot be aimed solely at the individual level without looking at the broader context (Maher, 1992).

The assumption that breastfeeding is merely a nutritional (or at most, psychological) matter lies behind both medical approaches and women's failure to take up a position with regard to these approaches. Breastfeeding, according to this assumption, is the same the world over – a matter of the 'successful' or 'unsuccessful' functioning of a physical or psychological relationship between two individuals. Yet breastfeeding involves much more than a relationship between individuals. The economic and social conditions of infant feeding have a fundamental effect on its chances of 'success'. Among these conditions are the extremely varied social and symbolic relationships which infant feeding creates and services in different cultures (Maher, 1992). The Northern Ireland mother's ability to choose to breastfeed, or to do so successfully, is equally influenced by the local culture. There is agreement among observers of the Northern Irish scene that 'above all else Ulster has been a religious region' (Akenson, 1973), indeed 'probably the most Christian society in the western world except for the Republic of Ireland' (Rose, 1971). Most observers have assumed that this means that Northern Ireland is different from the rest of the UK, if not the rest of Europe. One corollary of this difference is that people in Northern Ireland hold more authoritarian attitudes and values. It is within this context of deeply entrenched attitudes and values that mothers in Northern Ireland make choices about methods of infant feeding. Local research (Moss, 1990; Gordon, 1993) has clearly identified different cultural barriers to breastfeeding. With the cultural norm being bottle-feeding, a mother who chooses to breastfeed runs the risk of being unique, unusual and perhaps even rather deviant, especially if she decides to feed in a public place. The author (Gordon, 1993), when carrying out a recent research project exploring partners' attitudes to breastfeeding, recorded the following response when subjects were asked what type of woman they thought chose to breastfeed. Partners in favour of artificial feeding stated that they saw the breastfeeding mothers as self-confident and self-assertive, i.e. 'a woman with a wild lot of confidence', 'a forward sort o' girl – no shame in her' and 'showie weemen do it'. Partners with children being breastfed saw breastfeeding mothers as confident, caring and self-assertive. It is interesting to note the marked differences in how they perceived the mothers. The comments from fathers of formula-fed babies would definitely not have encouraged their wives to consider breastfeeding as an option. Embarrassment has also been shown to be a very real issue in relation to breastfeeding in Northern Ireland. Moss (1990) stated that mothers who breastfeed run the risk of being embarrassed or of embarrassing others. She also reported that it was socially unacceptable to breastfeed in public places, and partners reported varying degrees of embarrassment when their wives breastfed in front of family members or close friends.

The degree of freedom with which women are able to manage breastfeeding appears to depend on the configuration of roles which they are called upon to play in any given society. Partners', friends' and mothers' attitudes have also been shown to have a major influence on a woman's freedom to breastfeed in Northern Ireland. The research project carried out by the author in 1993 to investigate partners' attitudes to infant-feeding methods in County Antrim revealed that the attitudes of mothers to infant-feeding methods were often in agreement with their partners' wishes. Few societies appear to stress the duty of a father as a nurturer, yet in many societies it is the father who decides who shall breastfeed by whom, and for how long (Maher, 1992). In the Koran, within Islamic law, there is tremendous support and encouragement for breastfeeding. In Surat II, verse 233, in the Koran, it is stated that: 'The mothers shall give suck to their offsprings for two complete years, for those who desire to complete the term'. Within Islam, the mother has the duty to breastfeed and the father has the responsibility to provide an environment that facilitates breastfeeding for the 2-year period, unless they mutually decide to wean the child before the end of that period. This also includes provision for mother and child in the case of divorce, so that breastfeeding can continue, and the prohibition of wet-nursing where the mother is able to breastfeed herself. Breastfeeding is the norm, and is valued and supported by the family and Islamic community. In Maher's (1992) study of women in Morocco it is suggested, by contrast, that women turned to formula feeding as a way of gaining some control for themselves within a male-dominated society. An increase in the production of cash crops, rather than crops for their own consumption, meant that the men had financial control. By turning to formula feeds, the women were able to have legitimate access to some of the cash which their labour had produced. Breastfeeding meant no money and no control over their own lives. This provides us with some insight into the socio-economic factors which influence breastfeeding and reminds us that for many societies breastfeeding has more than a solely nutritional meaning. This illustrates the powerful influence that partners may exert on a mother's infant feeding within different cultures and the ramifications on a mother's feeding behaviour. Perhaps the attitudes of men in Northern Ireland are not as big an anomaly as was previously thought by the author when compared cross-culturally. However, this does not lessen the influence that partners may exert on a mother's infant feeding choice within the province. It would also appear that within Northern Ireland other members of the extended family can also have a strong influence on a mother's infant feeding choice. McKinley (1996), in a breastfeeding research project, carried out a survey of attitudes to breastfeeding and how breastfeeding should be promoted in the Southern Health Board (in County Armagh). It was found that participants over 65 years of age were most resistant both to the promotion of breastfeeding and to women breastfeeding in public. This age band includes mothers and grandmothers, a group already known from previous research to have a powerful influence on new mothers. Beske and Garvis (1982) found that the most frequently identified sources of discouragement were the maternal grandmother, the baby's father and the father's mother. The importance of support from individuals in a woman's social or kinship network for the success of breastfeeding has long been recognized (Dix, 1991; Alexy and Martin, 1994). Black (1980) claims that maternal attitudes towards breastfeeding must be consistent with the individual, family and social system goals if breastfeeding is to be attempted. In Northern Ireland, grandmothers have a strong influence on the extended family and on childrearing practices, as many also take on the role of child-minder when the mother returns to work. A multiplicity of factors therefore influence a mother's feeding choice in Northern Ireland, not only within the family arena but also as a result of the wider political issues, e.g. lack of maternity or paternity leave from work, unreasonable demands from employers, and last, but not least, the cultural taboos which deny the mother the right to breastfeed. It has been shown that the social factors which may affect rates of breastfeeding are proportional to mothers now returning to work, and the reduction in the availability of adequate maternity leave (Madden, 1987; Madlon-Kay, 1988). The responsibility for empowering a mother entails much more than giving her information, especially the well-worn rhetoric 'Breast is Best', now so familiar that its meaning may well be lost through familiarity. To empower mothers it is essential that health professionals themselves, first and foremost, are empowered if they are going to be able to help to remove some of the obstacles to breastfeeding within the cultural and/or political environment of Northern Ireland.

Essentially it is quality care that empowers women. This involves respect, acknowledgement of mothers' concerns within their own socio-economic groups, and the provision of sound scientific information that is understandable in terms sufficient to facilitate informed choice. It is essential to learn not only about physical needs but also about emotional and religious needs, so that the care offered is appropriate and sensitive to the mother's real needs. Empowerment is therefore a transactional concept involving a relationship with others – demands are nurtured by the effects of collaborative efforts (Keiffer, 1984).

Whilst advice and information are fundamental to empowerment, it is important to recognize that health professionals cannot empower mothers – it is mothers who empower themselves. Mothers need to be supported and given confidence in their own abilities. It is a social process of recognizing, promoting and enhancing people's ability to meet their own needs, solve their own problems, and mobilize the necessary resources in order to feel in control of their own lives (Gibson, 1991). Conflicting advice from health professionals has in the past often been directly opposed to what mothers instinctively wanted to do, when what was actually required was the development of collaborative partnerships in the use of resources and information that promoted a sense of control and self-efficacy. Similarly, hospitals laid down rules and routines rather than encouraging the mother herself to interpret the baby's behaviour and to assess her own and the baby's needs within the framework of their relationship and particular social circumstances.

One of the classic bases of power (French and Raven, 1959) is expert power, i.e. power founded on skills and knowledge. This gives nurses and midwives potentially, if not actually, powerful positions by virtue of their expertise. Whilst practitioners need this knowledge and these skills to be effective, they should not impose their expertise on clients, but instead use it as a tool for empowerment within the context of equal partnership with the client (Hess, 1984; Katz, 1984). Knowledge is gained from the collective sharing of experiences and understanding the social influences surrounding their lives (Wallerstein and Bernstein, 1988). Health care professionals need to give up control in order to help their clients to gain power. The instilling of confidence in a mother to enable her to breastfeed may rest not so much on her having more power but in her feeling more powerful – more enabled. The enhancement of her self-confidence is integral to her successful progress.

This may require professionals to surrender the need for control and be prepared to accept decisions different to those which had been previously decided for the mother. Professionals can wrongly feel a sense of having failed when a mother decides not to breastfeed, or opts to give up early. Success or failure should instead be measured from the level of quality care offered and the ability to facilitate informed choice, rather than the ultimate outcome. Health professionals have to start by helping mothers who really want to breastfeed in the first instance to ensure that these mothers achieve success.

Empowerment of professionals will require the unlearning of many traditional approaches, and re-examination of the nature of relationships with mothers, and the values and beliefs regarding their own professionalism which underpin them, developing new skills in negotiation, communication, facilitation and advocacy. To empower mothers, professionals need the self-confidence that stems from appropriate knowledge and expertise, and in particular they need self-awareness of their own feelings and prejudices stemming from perhaps a degree of enculturation within their own society. Mothers need to be given sufficient knowledge about the art of breastfeeding, specific benefits and inherent difficulties to enable them to trust their own knowledge, and to recognize that they can then make informed choices and can skilfully manage their infant feeding method of choice in a non-dependent manner.

The root of 'power' in the Latin *'potere'* is the ability to choose. Included in the dictionary definition are terms like 'enable' and 'permit'. Within Northern Ireland mothers also need the active support of professionals to help remove some of the obvious barriers to breastfeeding and give them the much needed 'permission' to choose it as an infant-feeding method when they so desire.

Empowering but a few more mothers to breastfeed could have the overall effect of changing attitudes within Northern Irish society. Although it has been shown that the larger structural (economic, political and cultural organization) forces in society shape the everyday lives of individuals, it is also true that the everyday practices of individuals can also shape some of the larger forces and bring about change.

Many epidemiological studies demonstrate the often profound role of poverty and other social, economic and political factors in influencing individual health status (Syme and Berkman, 1976; Black, 1980). Yet individuals have been able to re-shape the social context within which they live, and thus to affect their health. For example, disability rights groups such as the 'Independent Living Movement' have enabled people with disability to bring about great social changes to their benefit. There is therefore clearly interdependence between individual empowerment and empowerment at a more political level. Shor and Freire point out:

> While individual empowerment, the feeling of being changed, is not enough concerning the transformation of the whole society, it is absolutely necessary for the process of social transformation. The critical development of people is absolutely fundamental for the radical transformation of society ... but it is not enough by itself.
>
> (Shor and Freire, 1987, p. 6)

Empowerment can occur at many levels, from personal empowerment through community organizations to political action. Health professionals can empower at all of these levels, but different health professionals must work in partnership and use their different skills and knowledge to influence where they are most effective. Quality care given in the form of antenatal education and support to teenage mothers desiring to breastfeed is just as empowering as influencing health purchasers with regard to making provision for breastfeeding, or indeed becoming politically active to remove known barriers to breastfeeding – but all of these may be necessary to facilitate true and complete empowerment. Empowering those mothers who want to breastfeed to do so successfully may in fact be the catalyst required for many other mothers within Northern Ireland, through their ability to influence local attitudes and values and thus to bring about the necessary political changes that would better facilitate breastfeeding locally.

The challenges and changes to professional practice: the way forward in Northern Ireland

The Northern Board Breastfeeding Initiative Group was set up in 1991 to investigate possible strategies to promote breastfeeding locally. This multi-disciplinary group, which included representatives from the voluntary sector, was to become the power-house for many changes in relation to infant feeding. Faced with the stark reality of the first local Office of Population Censuses and Surveys results and evidence derived from local raw data, identifying Northern Ireland as having one of the lowest breastfeeding incidences in Europe, left the group in no doubt that significant initiatives were required to promote breastfeeding in the region. Concurrently, breastfeeding targets were being flagged up as part of health policy within a Government white paper, i.e. *The Health of the Nation* (Department of Health, 1991) in the UK, suggesting a targeted breastfeeding incidence of 75 per cent by 2000. This was mirrored in the Northern Ireland Regional Strategy (1992–1997), indicating an anticipated target rise from 29 per cent to 50 per cent breastfeeding incidence by 1997 (Department of Health and Social Services, Northern Ireland, 1992).

A multidisciplinary subgroup set to the task of producing research-based breastfeeding guidelines for circulation to all key health professionals who had contact with antenatal and postnatal mothers. Draft circulation of the document clearly revealed evidence of some lack of breastfeeding knowledge and skills, and unfortunately, as suspected, the existence of the age-old problem of conflicting advice. It was realized from the outset that such guidelines would not be adequate on their own to change breastfeeding practice, since an excellent research-based text, *Successful Breast Feeding* had been issued to all midwives in 1988, but sadly there has been little real evidence of its application. The newly published breastfeeding guidelines were disseminated to all health professionals, including GPs in contact with mothers, in the hope that local ownership would help to refocus health professionals to make real use of them and to ensure that scientific evidence was applied to practice. A second working group set to the task of critiquing the available breastfeeding promotional leaflets and materials, and investigated the production of more suitable materials for use locally. This led to the production of two breastfeeding leaflets available for use by all health professionals with the intention of removing dependence on promotional materials produced by milk companies. Only these and a leaflet produced by the Health Promotion Agency were recommended for use in the Northern Board Area.

It was recognized by the Breastfeeding Initiative Group that some form of breastfeeding awareness training or update was also necessary to empower health professionals if they were to become more effective in helping more mothers to breastfeed successfully.

An educational package relevant to local health professionals appeared to be the first necessary step in creating an environment that was conducive to successful breastfeeding. Becker (1992), in a study carried out in rural maternity units in Ireland to ascertain the levels of breastfeeding knowledge among hospital staff, found rising breastfeeding rates in the units where midwives were more recently qualified and had higher knowledge scores.

A local *Breastfeeding Training Manual* compiled by the author was strongly influenced by clinical practitioners representing health visitors, midwives, dietitians and health promotion, and also by publications from the Baby-Friendly Initiative. The UNICEF documents set out the global criteria for a 'Baby-Friendly Initiative' with the '10 steps to successful breastfeeding'. These were the ideal quality standards which the Breastfeeding Initiative Group hoped to strive towards and achieve, both in the hospital and in the community. This was not an attempt to convert all mothers to breastfeeding, but instead to ensure that those mothers who wanted to breastfeed were facilitated and enabled to do so successfully. The training package involved 5 half study days and was intended for health visitors, midwives and paediatric nurses working together in multidisciplinary groups. Negotiations with the College of Midwifery in Belfast resulted in 12 key personnel being offered places on a course called 'Breastfeeding Management and Promotion' to prepare further a group of local trainers. This group was again multidisciplinary and included in its membership midwives, health visitors and a Health Promotion Officer.

Completion of this training coincided with a 'fact-finding' day in London run by the combined efforts of the Health Visitors Association and the Royal College of Midwives to investigate the possibility of creating an 'Invest in Breast Together' trainers' course. This timely intervention offered the Northern Ireland group the opportunity to build on and, to some extent, reshape some of the work already completed locally. The author, a health visitor, partnered by a midwifery colleague, represented Northern Ireland at these fact-finding days, and presented the details of the training manual produced in Northern Ireland. This multidisciplinary forum explored all of the identified needs in relation to breastfeeding training and provided the backdrop necessary to start the work on a training pack suitable for preparing expert trainers across the UK. The aim of the 'Invest in Breast Together' training was to produce expert trainers who would cascade knowledge to fellow practitioners either through actual training or by role-modelling good practice.

Training had already commenced by this stage in four sites across the Northern Board Area using the locally produced breastfeeding training manual. A health visitor and midwife combined their training efforts with local dietitians and National Childbirth Trust members. The trainees were drawn from health visiting, midwifery and paediatric nursing, and ensured a good cross-section of experience at each session.

The final pioneering 'Invest in Breast Together' training package (Kendall,

1995) also used multidisciplinary peer training, but focused more on addressing attitudes, values and perceptions rather than simply technique. The evolution of such a course for Northern Ireland trainers at this time was very exciting, as it was the missing dimension locally. It dovetailed perfectly with the locally produced training manual as a tool to train trainers, and gave the autonomy necessary to provide a complete programme of peer training for multidisciplinary groups within the Northern Health Board. A large breastfeeding conference, hosted by the Northern Health Board and the DHSS, launched both the training packs and the Breastfeeding Initiative in Northern Ireland with delegates drawn from all of the four Health Boards across the province and also some representatives from Southern Ireland. Wide media coverage was captured using local press, television and radio reports. As a consequence, representatives from all the other three Health Board Areas attended training, thus providing key breastfeeding trainers ready for the task of cascading training within their own Health Board Areas.

The UK approach to breastfeeding

The overarching principle of Invest in Breast was to empower women to initiate and continue breastfeeding through empowering health professionals to support them more effectively in their efforts. Partnership is an essential component of empowering – thus the main aim of the training was to create an environment of trust, partnership and informative guidance between health professionals and mothers, and among health professionals themselves. The training focuses on skills of reflection and facilitation, utilization of research-based evidence to inform practice, and communication skills, and draws on practitioners' own experiences. The Invest in Breast training provided an ideal opportunity to address attitudes and values, rather than simply dealing with breastfeeding technique.

It was critically important that any training programme addressed not just skills and knowledge but also attitudes, beliefs and values, aware that local researchers had shown the potential impact of negative attitudes on breastfeeding practice. Within Northern Ireland this would be no easy task, in view of the fact that Northern Irish people were known for their very fixed attitudes, values and belief systems (Akenson, 1973).

One such negative attitude was reported by McKnight (1987), who stated in research conducted in Belfast that, whilst many health professionals did believe that breast milk was good, sadly some allowed themselves to believe that formula milk was just as good – whilst very subtle, this is one of the most dangerous attitudes with regard to promoting breastfeeding. Some professionals also reported concern about creating guilt in mothers who had chosen not to breastfeed, resulting in the development of *laissez-faire* or passive attitudes by health professionals with regard to promoting breast-feeding as a method of infant feeding, lest they offend. Empowerment is about information and choice, but essentially informed choice where the health professionals are enabled to present all the accurate research-based evidence, and to present all of the options available to each mother within a relationship of partnership, and with relevance to the mother's socio-economic and cultural background.

Learning to learn and empowering professionals

The theoretical underpinning of any form of training had to be that of androgogy as described by Knowles (1990), who identified the following five areas in which he believed adults were unique as learners: the concept of the learner; the role of the learner's experience; the learner's readiness to learn; the learner's orientation to learning; and finally the learner's motivation to learn. These health professionals did not come to the training as empty vessels, but as critical thinking and inspiring adults bringing with them a richness of experience which needed to be shared to enable themselves and the rest of the groups to grow and benefit from each other's breastfeeding knowledge and skills. In fact, many Northern Irish practitioners would have been alienated by the thought of professionals requiring further breast-feeding training. The philosophy was therefore one of professional partner-ship and collaboration.

Several factors had to exist within the training for empowerment to occur. Primarily, this required creation of a caring environment in which trust, honesty, openness and genuineness could develop. This was to facilitate two-way communication between the trainer and trainees to ensure the development of trust and empowerment, and to emphasize that partner-ships, contributions and breastfeeding experiences were valued and shared by the whole group. Planning together and setting joint learning objectives ensured that the group in its entirety had a shared purpose and vision, and that quite early on there was evidence of commitment and ownership from within the group.

The educational approach involved a shift from trainers as instructors (Gagne, 1975) to trainers as facilitators (Rogers, 1989), i.e. individuals who enable practitioners to explore and discover, discuss and share rather than simply convey information. This required the skills necessary to create conversations with participants to enable them to look at breastfeeding practices and ask what they meant for themselves and for clients, for theory and practice, and for shared understanding and developing of knowledge. This proved to be a much more demanding task than had previously been realized, necessitating real use of facilitative skills, active listening, and learning to move back and use 'teaching moments' as the group provided them in a rich learning environment for everyone.

An important inherent assumption of this training pack was that adults learn through experience, as proposed through the work of Schon (1983) and Mezirow (1981).

The pack draws upon these ideas to enable practitioners to learn through experience by developing reflective and analytical skills. These techniques value experiential learning and the wealth of rich experience which many practitioners brought to the course. It did assume that participants had previous breastfeeding knowledge and the experience and skills necessary to support breastfeeding mothers. The expectation was that these breastfeeding trainers would emerge not only as knowledgeable 'do-ers', but also as expert role models with increased communicative and facilitative training skills. The reflective component within the 'Invest in Breast' training was a new addition to local training, and the pre-course material included a requirement to keep a reflective journal with the theme of reflecting on practice flowing throughout the entire course both for trainers and for trainees.

This proved to be an exciting and valuable addition because the reflective practice became a window on the subtlety and complexity of practices, and helped to illuminate deficiencies where these were present. Kolb (1984) defined learning as a process whereby knowledge is created through transformation of experience. He emphasized the need for any educational activity to engage the learner in a continuous and alternating process of investigation and exploration, followed by reflection. Kolb believed knowledge to be continuously modified with experience. Acquiring new knowledge and skills and modifying practice is a life-long process for all accountable health professionals. Planned reflection proved to be both insightful and self-regulating for the breastfeeding trainees and trainers, when considering their practice. Street (1991) described reflection as a way to empower nurses to become fully cognizant of their own knowledge and actions, the personal and professional histories which have shaped them, the symbols and images inherent in the language they use, the myths and the metaphors which constrain them in practice, their nursing experiences, and the potentialities and constraints of their work setting.

The participants consolidated the concepts of reflective practice by means of critical incident analysis and problem-solving techniques using issues from their reflective journals. Considerable interaction resulted, with a substantial volume of both knowledge and research being spontaneously provided from within the groups. This combined individual reflective skills with focus participative group reflection. The trainers were also challenged to reflect continually on their facilitative skills and training technique during the entire course, and shared reflective moments in partnership with the trainees to evaluate the teaching/learning response. Role modelling emphasized the value of shared reflection for all aspects of practice, including training. This helped to engender true partnership throughout the entire training process.

A model for empowering professionals

At the beginning of the 5-day training course the concepts of partnership and empowerment were fully explored in an exercise, as these were integral to the whole philosophy underpinning the training process. This exercise afforded the opportunity to discuss experiences and interpretations of the terms within the groups, and thus to explore positive and negative feelings about partnership and empowerment. This proved to be a very necessary exercise because initially partnership was obviously inhibited until participants became more aware of the value of each other's unique contributions in supporting breastfeeding mothers. It was apparent (from the training) that 'little box mentalities' did still exist among some health professionals, and concerted efforts were required to allow practitioners to debrief before the real working together and environment of trust could exist. It was disappointing to observe some practitioners' negative reactions to peer training and to the valuable role played by the voluntary group representatives. In the NHS today there is clearly much focus on professionals working together and inter-agency work to provide a needs-led, seamless service, and the UKCC Code of Conduct number 6 (1992) holds nurses accountable to work in partnership where it states that 'work in a collaborative and co-operative manner with health care professionals and other agencies in providing care, and recognize their particular contributions within the care team.'

Role modelling of a trainer partnership (using a health visitor and a midwife working together as joint trainers) proved most beneficial throughout, as it gave an overt lead to the practitioners.

Salvage (1990) argues that the ideology of partnership is at the root of a fundamental reform movement in UK nursing: the 'new nursing'. A therapeutic nurse–patient relationship is implied, based on mutual respect, trust and equality of worth. Such a relationship is fundamental to a mother making an informed choice with regard to infant-feeding method. Equally important is professional partnership if mothers are to be offered the necessary seamless support to help them to succeed in their efforts to breastfeed. Small groups of nurses drawn from different specialisms, but practising in the same location, worked together on course projects. This also engendered partnership, and as these projects produced some excellent innovative ideas to take back to practice, it was evident that these partnerships would continue long after the training ceased.

Invest in Breast offered several unique exercises within the training pack which proved to be very significant for empowering health professionals in Northern Ireland, in particular exploring attitudes and values, cultural issues, and organizing change.

Exercises on attitudes and values proved particularly valuable, as these involved an activity requiring participants to reflect on pictures of women ranging from 'page 3' models to breastfeeding mothers. This revealed clear evidence of conservative attitudes and reservations openly displayed by many health professionals locally as they viewed the images of the naked breasts, and sadly these same reactions may also have influenced their views on mothers breastfeeding in public. This proved an important activity in highlighting to the participants the possible detrimental effect of demonstrating such negative attitudes. Unfortunately it was evident from the exercise that some health professionals also found feeding in public embarrassing and openly disapproved of the practice. Viewing and comparing attitude scales relating to breastfeeding also proved thought-provoking for many participants, as it provided evidence of erroneous ideas, false presumptions and identified preconceived notions about the types of mothers who breastfeed. Both the use of the pictures and attitude scales provided excellent tools to enable participants to explore their own attitudes openly, share them and later reflect on them. This was a very novel way to view attitudes and values in the group setting, and many Northern Ireland health professionals appeared to be surprised by their own negative and conservative views when exposed to the group as a whole. Reflecting honestly on attitudes in an environment of trust where openness and genuineness developed proved to be a valuable learning experience for both trainers and trainees, and all were enthusiastic to share this illuminating experience with their colleagues.

This exercise was very significant in view of the fact that Dix (1991) had reported that influencing factors in the decision to bottle-feed were negative attitudes towards breastfeeding. Local researchers (McKnight, 1987; Murray and Webster, 1988) had also reported that these negative attitudes did exist among some Northern Irish health professionals as well as among other members of society. Heightening the awareness of negative attitudes was the first step in attempting to change them, especially when they are exposed through personal and group reflection and then critically analysed. No previous breastfeeding training had attempted such a technique, and its value was self-evident in the quality of the group work which ensued. An exercise focusing on cultural differences was also particularly pertinent to practitioners in Northern Ireland where, as already stated, it is culturally correct to bottle-feed. Participants reflected on the power of cultural influence and explored the potential conflict in relation to cultural variation, exposing the inherent difficulties placed in the way of mothers wishing to choose breastfeeding as their infant-feeding method.

Over half a day's activity was also spent on the theory and practice of change. With the use of case studies and personal accounts of change within their own organization, participants discussed the most effective methods of managing change in the light of their personal experiences. This was also an important exercise considering that managing change in practice would be a necessary component in both hospital and community in order to facilitate and better support breastfeeding mothers. The breastfeeding trainers were returning to practice as change agents, and this exercise gave insight into how best to initiate lasting and effective change.

Focus groups reflecting together on experiences and problem-solving provided a rich learning environment in which knowledge and skills from within the groups were used to maximum effect. When working together to critique research, not only was there a heightened awareness of research-based practice, but also a natural sharing of research articles among participants. Informal support networks among practitioners were evidenced. Presentations and project work generated shared, innovative ideas that were ready to be translated back into practice.

The effectiveness of breastfeeding training – are health professionals and mothers in Northern Ireland empowered?

The third year of training has now commenced within the Northern Board, and it is envisaged that all midwives, health visitors and neonatal nurses will have completed the training by the end of 1998. This training has also been cascaded in two of the three other Health Boards with a network of expert trainers established within all of Northern Ireland's Provider Trusts to maintain the ongoing breastfeeding work.

Breastfeeding training seminars have also been provided for local general practitioners and their trainees in order to ensure a multidisciplinary approach and a shared vision for breastfeeding mothers within primary care. Breastfeeding study days and conferences have increased across all four Health Boards, resulting in evidence of increased interest in the need to promote breastfeeding. Commissioners within the Northern Board have worked in partnership with local expert trainers to formulate a breastfeeding strategy action plan which has been issued to all of its provider units. This ensures that quality standards set within the training are mirror-imaged into the contracting process which, in turn, defines the quality of service. The Department of Health and Social Services sponsored a 1-day conference to assimilate all of the ongoing initiatives within Northern Ireland and have set up a breastfeeding group at Department level to facilitate and support local efforts to meet regional breastfeeding targets by the year 2002.

One significant increase in breastfeeding incidence has been clearly demonstrated in a large maternity unit in Belfast in 1996, where the incidence increased by 8 per cent following a local training initiative. The entire hospital staff, including nurse managers, were offered a 2-day breastfeeding training course planned locally. The in-house training was completed comparatively quickly, with these remarkable results, demonstrating the effectiveness of targeting an entire maternity unit with its accompanying community staff in order to bring about change.

The process of empowering health professionals through breastfeeding training is now well established across Northern Ireland. There is certainly a heightened awareness of the importance of breastfeeding in Northern Ireland, but much still needs to be done to accelerate the process. Hospital practices are being audited and critically reviewed, and many could now claim to be achieving at least some of the '10 steps to successful breastfeeding' of the Baby-Friendly Initiatives (UNICEF and World Health Organization, 1989). As a result, formulation of Breastfeeding Policies has set out clearly the same set of principles for all staff to adhere to, and so minimizes the tendency for new mothers to receive conflicting advice. Monitoring staff compliance with breastfeeding intention and outcome has therefore become a routine part of the audit cycle. Several large hospitals are striving to achieve at least some of the requisite stages to become Baby-Friendly. Sadly, no hospital in Northern Ireland at present could aspire to a 75 per cent incidence of breastfeeding, which is the prerequisite for Baby-Friendly status. However, one maternity unit in East Belfast has been successful in achieving a 'certificate of commitment' in a staged plan to become the first 'Baby-Friendly' hospital in Northern Ireland.

As a result of these changes, more babies are able to have skin contact with their mothers within the first hour following birth, and 'rooming-in' occurs in most units. Early mother–infant contact serves the infant by securing maternal attachment (Gubernick, 1981). This is a biological imperative and deserves to be a core practice of intrapartum care irrespective of how the mother chooses to feed her infant. Some maternity units have now started to place breastfeeding mothers together in wards where they are more easily supported, so encouraging peer support, and 'bedding-in' is no longer an unfamiliar sight in some units. A Mid-Ulster maternity unit is piloting the use of a mother-held feeding record indicative of a real partnership approach in recording all advice sought and offered to the new mother with regard to infant feeding. This card was produced by a midwife and a health visitor as part of their Invest in Breast project work.

The custom of giving breastfeeding babies complementary feeds of formula milk has been particularly discouraged throughout the training, and a decrease has been reported from 45 per cent in 1990 to 36 per cent in 1995 (Foster *et al.*, 1997). This is a significant achievement considering such feeds have been shown to be associated with early termination of breastfeeding (White *et al.*, 1992). Cup-feeding has become a much more familiar sight in some neonatal units; cup or spoon feeds can safely overcome the problem of giving complementary feeds where they are medically indicated (Lang *et al.*, 1994). Cup-feeding has been successfully introduced in some units and appears to be associated with a greater success rate for establishing breastfeeding. There has been a greater provision of both hand and electric breast pumps for mothers' use both in hospitals and in the community. Sadly, infant formula is still sold in some Child Health Clinics in the province, and milk companies continue to make an impact with their advertising campaigns, still attempting to bribe health professionals to influence mothers' choices indirectly. Hopefully better informed health professionals and better informed mothers will become much more discerning about the marketing tactics of milk companies.

There is no doubt that some visible changes with regard to infant feeding have taken place in Northern Ireland. Health professionals have produced local breastfeeding policies and written quality standards relating to breastfeeding management and promotion. These have not been allowed simply to become paper exercises, but instead have been audited to ensure that quality is maintained by peer audit and management review, both of which include consumer opinions.

Parents in general have also become much more aware of their rights and in particular, the consumer voice for mothers has been strengthened because of policies such as 'Changing Childbirth'. The inclusion of representatives from breastfeeding voluntary groups within planning and breastfeeding training has also meant that professionals are being challenged more frequently about the quality of services being offered to all mothers. Whilst much certainly appears to have improved in relation to promoting and managing breastfeeding locally it is the most recent Office for National Statistics (Foster *et al.*, 1997) results which have provided the first real evidence of changes having taken place in infant-feeding choices in Northern Ireland (see Table 8.1).

Table 8.1 Incidence of breastfeeding by country

Year	England/Wales	Scotland	Northern Ireland
1990	64%	50%	36%
1995	68%	55%	45%

The most significant change in breastfeeding incidence has occurred in Northern Ireland when compared to England, Wales and Scotland, with an increase of 9 per cent from 36 per cent in 1990 to 45 per cent in 1995. This is almost twice the increase shown in any of the other UK countries. Whilst this is an indication that the training programme may have been successful in empowering more professionals and mothers, it would be difficult to state this conclusively. It begs the question of whether things were beginning to change in Northern Ireland anyway, and how much of this success can actually be correlated with this new empowering approach to training. It is also possible that the flagging up of regional breastfeeding targets as part of health strategies could have been the impetus required to motivate more health professionals actively to promote breastfeeding and to manage it more effectively.

Whilst acceptance or rejection of breastfeeding has been influenced in the western world to some extent by the knowledge of human lactation, sadly cultural rejection, negative attitudes, and lack of support from health professionals still exist and, to some degree, are hindering it in Northern Ireland. The breastfeeding training programme addressed these issues in particular by challenging negative attitudes, and at the same time it attempted to empower professionals with the requisite skills in order to provide more effective support and encouragement to ensure lactation success and adherence to health care guidelines. Combining training efforts with voluntary groups, i.e. La Leche and National Childbirth Trust representatives, has also contributed greatly to the initiative because these groups have already been recognized for the success of their mother-to-mother programmes. This provides an excellent example of how the power of positive peer relationships can be utilized to counteract, at least in part, unhelpful or negative social relationships where they do exist within communities or family units.

Certainly training has heightened awareness and increased professional focus on breastfeeding, and has been the catalyst that has caused many changes in practice. These quantitative results provide some tangible evidence of success, but they also highlight the need at this time of current change for a thorough evaluation study to investigate fully which other factors may also have influenced the decision of more mothers to breastfeed. Therein may lie more evidence which will further empower health professionals to support mothers fully in their infant-feeding choice.

Conclusions

The real work of change in Northern Ireland has begun, and the attitudes of both health professionals and the public are being challenged. Scientific evidence continues to reinforce the health benefits of breastfeeding for both mother and baby, but many political issues with regard to employment and lack of facilities for breastfeeding mothers locally still need to be addressed. The Government now recognizes the value of the breastfeeding resource in relation to health gain, and has provided the targets to be achieved into the next millennium. Perhaps it will be empowered Northern Ireland mothers wishing to breastfeed who will bring about the greatest change through the consumer voice.

Health professional skills are being honed to better prepare them both to promote and to support breastfeeding mothers more effectively not only in hospitals and the community, but also in society in general. However, empowering mothers to breastfeed, is a process that requires the efforts of everyone in society. It requires commitment on the part of the health care institutions, decision-makers and government, to name but a few. They need supportive homes, health care facilities and work environments. This means having access to accurate information and communicating their needs to their families, health care providers and employers.

Merely telling women to breastfeed or acknowledging their right to do so, whilst not removing the obstacles and ensuring that they receive the necessary support to breastfeed, is not empowering. Much still needs to be done in the Northern Ireland context if it is to be nurtured back to a breastfeeding culture. The health gains have been annotated, the difficulties and barriers illuminated, and now there are planned attempts to bring about real change for mothers and babies in Northern Ireland.

It is clear that breastfeeding is more difficult for women in Northern Ireland today because of their economic role, lack of informal societal breastfeeding support systems, and the erotic perception of breasts. Health professionals will have to continue to assist children, young people, and adult men and women to see breastfeeding as a normal function which persists for more than a week or two, and happens outside as well as inside the home. Moreover, the 'education' of health professionals about breastfeeding must be strengthened, and continued. A consistent, persistent, supportive approach is essential if attitudes and behaviour are to change in Northern Ireland. Whilst local health professionals are but part of the resolution to the low incidence of breastfeeding, they are nevertheless accountable for their actions and cannot abdicate their responsibilities with regard to the health of their nation and/or their future generation.

References

Akenson, D.H. 1973: *Education and enmity: the control of schooling in Northern Ireland 1920–50.* Newton Abbot: David and Charles.

Alexy, B. and Martin, A.C. 1994: Breastfeeding: perceived barriers and benefits/enhancers in a rural and urban setting. *Public Health Nursing* 11, 214–18.

American Academy of Paediatrics 1982: Nutrition Committee of the Canadian Paediatric Society and the Committee on Nutrition of the American Academy of Pediatrics. Breast-Feeding – a Commentary in Celebration of the International Year of the Child. *Breast Feeding Paediatrics* 62, 591–600.

Backett, K. 1992: The construction of health knowledge in middle-class families. *Health Education Research* 7, 497–506.

Baucher, H., Laventhal, J.M. and Shapiroz, E.D. 1986: Studies of breast feeding and infections: how good is the evidence? *Journal of the American Medical Association* 256, 887–92.

Becker, G.E. 1992: Breastfeeding knowledge of hospital staff in rural maternity units in Ireland. *Journal of Human Lactation* 8, 137–42.

Beske, J. and Garvis, M. 1982: Important factors in breastfeeding success. *American Journal of Maternal–Child Nursing* 7, 174–8.

Black, D. 1980: *Inequalities in health. Report of a research working party.* London: Department of Health and Social Security (chairman Sir Douglas Black).

Black, R., Blair, J., Jones, V. and Durant, R. 1990: Infant feeding decisions among pregnant women from a WIC population in Georgia. *Journal of the American Dietetic Association* **90**, 250–9.

Blair, H. 1977: Natural history of childhood asthma. *Archives of Disease in Childhood* **52**, 613–19.

Brunn, S. 1986: Grass-roots support for breastfeeding. *World Health Forum* **7**, 65–8.

Burne, S.R. 1976: Breast feeding. *Lancet* **2**, 261.

Burr, M. 1989: Environment factors and symptoms in infants at high risk of allergy. *Journal of Epidemiology and Community Health*, **43**: 125–32.

Butterfield, P. 1990: Thinking upstream: nurturing a conceptual understanding of the societal context of health behaviour. *Advances in Nursing Science* **12**, 1–8.

Calnan, M. 1986: Maintaining health and preventing illness: a comparison of the perception of women from different social classes. *Health Promotion* **1**, 167–77.

Cole, J. 1977: Breastfeeding in the Boston suburbs in relation to personal–social factors. *Clinical Pediatrics* **16**, 352–6.

Countryman, B.A. 1973: Breast care in the early puerperium. *Journal of Obstetric, Gynaecologic and Neonatal Nursing* **2**, 36–40.

Crawford, M.A. 1993: The role of essential fatty acids in neural development: implications for perinatal nutrition. *American Journal of Clinical Nutrition* **57** (Suppl.), 703S-710S.

Cunningham, A.S. 1987: Breast feeding is protective. *Paediatrics* **79**, 1052–3.

Department of Health 1991: *The Health of the Nation*. London: HMSO.

Department of Health 1993: *Changing childbirth* (the Report of the Expert Maternity Group). London: HMSO.

Department of Health 1994: Weaning and the weaning diet. *Report on Health and Social Subjects* No. 45. London: HMSO.

Department of Health and Social Services, Northern Ireland 1992: *A Regional Strategy for Northern Ireland, 1992–1997*. Belfast, HMSO.

Dix, D.N. 1991: Why women decide not to breastfeed. *Birth* **18**, 222–5.

Dumas, K., Pakter, J. and Krongrad, E. 1988: Postnatal medical and epidemiological risk factors for the sudden infant death syndrome. In Harper, R.M. and Hoffman, H.J. (eds), *Sudden infant death syndrome*. New York: PMA Publishing Corporation.

Duncan, B. and Holberg, E.J. 1993: Exclusive breast feeding for at least 4 months protects against otitis media. *Paediatrics* **91**, 867–72.

Facione, N. 1990: Otitis media: an overview of acute and chronic disease. *Nurse Practitioner* **15**, 11–22.

Fahlberg, L.L., Poulin, A.L., Girdano, D.A. and Dusek, D.E. 1991: Empowerment as an emerging approach to health education. *Journal of the Institute of Health Education* **22**, 185–93.

Farquharson, J. 1995: Effect of diet on the fatty acid composition of the major phospholipids of infant cerebral cortex. *Archives of Disease in Childhood* **72**, 198–203.

Feinstein, A.R. 1985: *Clinical epidemiology: the architecture of clinical research*. Philadelphia, W.B. Saunders Co., 683–718.

Foster, K., Lader, D. and Chessbrough, S. 1997: *Infant Feeding 1995. Office for National Statistics*. London: The Stationery Office.

French, J.R.P. and Raven, B. 1959: The bases of social power. In Cartwright, D. (ed.), *Studies in social power*. Chelsea, MI: Ann Arbor Press, 150–67.

Gagne, R. 1975: *Essentials of learning for instruction*. Hindale, IL: The Dryden Press.

Gibson, C.H. 1991: A conceptual analysis of empowerment. *Journal of Advanced Nursing* **16**, 354–61.

Goldman, A.S. 1993: The immune system of human milk: anti-microbial, anti-inflammatory, and immunomodulating properties. *Paediatric Infectious Disease Journal* **12**, 664–71.

Gordon, M.R. 1993: *An exploration of fathers' opinions of infant feeding method in Co. Antrim.* Unpublished paper, Department of Nursing and Health Visiting, University of Ulster.

Greco, L., Auficchio, S. and Mayer, M. 1988: Case-controlled study on nutritional risk factors in coeliac disease. *Journal of Paediatric Gastroenterology and Nutrition* **7**, 395–9.

Grulee, C.G., Sanford, H.N. and Schwartz, H. 1986: Breast and artificially fed infants. *Journal of the American Medical Association* **104**, 1935.

Gubernick, D.J. 1981: Parent and infant attachment in mammals. In Gubernick, D.J. and Klopfer, P.H. (eds), *Parental care in mammals.* New York: Plenum Press, 243–305.

Hess, R. 1984: Thoughts on empowerment. *Prevention in Human Sciences* **3**, 227–30.

Horwitz, R.I. and Feinstein, A.R. 1979: Methodologic standards and contradictory results in case-control research. *American Journal of Medicine* **66**, 556–63.

House of Commons Select Committee on Health 1992: *Second Report: Maternity Services (the Winterton report).* London: HMSO.

Howie, P.W. and Forsyth, J.S. 1990: Protective effect of breast-feeding against infection. *British Medical Journal* **300**, 11–16.

Jones, D.A. 1986: Attitudes of breastfeeding mothers: a survey of 647 mothers. *Social Science Medicine* **23**, 1151–6. .

Kalezko, S., Sherman, P., Corey, M. *et al.* 1989: Role of infant feeding practices in development of Crohn's disease in childhood. *British Medical Journal* **298**, 1617–18.

Kalnins, I. 1992: Children, empowerment and health promotion: some new directions in research and practice. *Health Promotion International* **7**, 53–9.

Kassianos, G. 1993: Promoting breastfeeding in the community. *Modern Midwife* **3**, 24–5.

Katz, R. 1984: Empowerment and synergy: expanding the community's healing resources. *Prevention in Human Sciences* **3**, 201–26.

Keiffer, C. 1984: Citizen empowerment: a developmental perspective. *Prevention in Human Sciences* **3**, 9–36.

Kendall, S. 1995: Cross-cultural aspects and breastfeeding promotion. *Health Visitor* **68**, 450–51.

Kitzinger, S. 1994: *Breastfeeding your baby.* London: Dorling Kindersley.

Knaft, K. 1974: Conflicting perspectives on breastfeeding. *American Journal of Nursing* **74**, 1848–951.

Knowles, M. 1990: *The adult learner: a neglected species,* 4th edn. Houston, TX: Gulf Publishing Co.

Kolb, D.A. 1984: *Experimental learning: experience as the source of learning and development.* Englewood Cliffs, NJ: Prentice-Hall.

Lang, S., Lawrence, C.J. and Orme, R. l'E. 1994: Cup feeding: an alternative method of infant feeding. *Archives of Disease in Childhood* **71**, 365–9.

Lanting, C.L. 1994: Neurological differences between nine-year-old children fed breast milk or formula milk as babies. *Lancet* **344**, 1319–22.

Lucas, A., Morley, R. and Cole, T.J. 1992: Breast milk and subsequent intelligence quotient in children born pre-term. *Lancet* **339**, 261–4.

McKinley, M. 1996: *A survey of attitudes to breastfeeding and how it should be promoted.* School of Biological and Biomedical Sciences, Faculty of Science, University of Ulster, Ulster.

McKnight, A. 1987: Breastfeeding: more than just health education. *Midwife, Health Visitor and Community Nurse* **23**, 302–12.

Madden, B.R. 1987: Breastfeeding and the working mother. *Journal of Public Health Policy* **8**, 531–41.

Madlon-Kay, D.J. 1988: Effect of decreasing maternity leave on breastfeeding. *Family Medicine* **20**, 220–1.

Maher, V. (ed.) 1992: *The anthropology of breastfeeding*, 5th edn. Oxford: Berg.

Metcalf, M.A. and Baum, J.D. 1992: Family characteristics and insulin-dependent diabetes. *Archives of Disease in Childhood* **67**, 731–6.

Mezirow, J. 1981: A critical theory of adult learning and education. *Adult Education* **32**, 3–24.

Michin, M. 1985: Breastfeeding matters. In Royal College of Midwives (ed.), *Successful breastfeeding. A practical guide for midwives*, 2nd edn. London: Churchill Livingstone, xi.

Mitchell, E.A., Scragg, R. and Stewart, A.W. 1991: Cot death supplement: results from the first year of the New Zealand Cot Death Study. *New Zealand Medical Journal* **104**, 71.

Mok, J. 1993: Breast milk and HIV-I transmission. *Lancet* **341**, 930–1.

Morgan, E. 1985: *The descent of woman*. London: Souvenir Press.

Morley, R. and Cole, T.J. 1988: Mothers' choice to provide breast milk and developmental outcomes. *Archives of Disease in Childhood* **63**, 1382–5.

Moss, R. 1990: *Breastfeeding in a bottle-feeding world*. Ulster: Faculty of Social Science and Health Sciences, University of Ulster.

Murray, P.S. and Webster, B. 1988: *Infant feeding in Derry and Oxford. Centre for Applied Health Studies*, University of Ulster, Centre for Applied Health Studies.

Niven, C. 1992: *Psychological care for families before, during and after birth*. Oxford: Butterworth-Heinemann.

Palmer, G. 1993a: *The politics of breast feeding*. London: Pandora Press.

Palmer, G. 1993b: Who helps health professionals with breastfeeding? *Midwives' Chronicle* **106**, 147–56.

Patterson, E. 1994: A case-control investigation of perinatal risk factors for childhood. IDDM in Northern Ireland and Scotland. *Diabetic Care* **17**, 376–81.

Pisacane, A. 1990: Breast feeding and urinary tract infection. *Lancet* **336**, 50.

Pisacane, A. 1994: Breast feeding and acute lower respiratory infection. *Acta Paediatrica* **83**, 8–14.

Pisacane, A. 1995: Breast feeding and acute appendicitis. *British Medical Journal* **310**, 836–7.

Pisacane, A., Impagliazzo, N. and De Caprio, C. 1996: Breast-feeding and tonsillectomy. *British Medical Journal* **312**, 746–7.

Rajan, L. 1993: The contribution of professional support, information and consistent correct advice to successful breast feeding. *Midwifery* **9**, 197–209.

Rappaport, J. 1984: Studies in empowerment: introduction to the issue. *Prevention in Human Services* **3**, 1–7.

Rogers, J. 1989: *Adults learning*, 3rd edn. Milton Keynes: Open University Press.

Rose, R. 1971: *Governing without consensus: an Irish Perspective*. London: Faber and Faber.

Saarinen, U. and Kajoasaari, M. 1995: Breastfeeding as prophylaxis against atopic disease: prospective follow-up study until 17 years old. *Lancet* **346**, 1065–9.

Salvage, J. 1990: The theory and practice of the 'new nursing'. *Nursing Times* **86**, 42–5.

Savage, F. 1992: Breast feeding – S.I.D.S. *Midirs Midwifery Digest* **2**, 3–5.

Schon, D.A. 1983: *The reflective practitioner: how professionals think in action*. New York: Basic Books.

Shelton, K. 1994: Empowering women to breastfeed successfully. *Breastfeeding Review* **2**, 455–8.

Shor, I. and Freire, P. 1987: *A pedagogy for liberation: dialogues on transforming education*. South Hadley, MA: Begin & Garvey.

Sloper, K., McKean, L. and Baum, J.D. 1974: Patterns of infant feeding in Oxford. *Archives of Disease in Childhood* **49**, 749.

Soni, J. 1988: Saved by the bottle. *Community Outlook*, 9 March 1988 (Insert in *Nursing Times* **84**, 10–14).

Street, A. 1991: *From image to action – reflection in nursing practice*. Geelong, Victoria: Deakin University Press.

Syme, S.L. and Berkman, L.F. 1976: Social class, susceptibility and sickness. *American Journal of Epidemiology* **104**, 1–8.

Thiry, L. 1985: Isolation of AIDS virus from cell-free breast milk of three healthy virus carriers. *Lancet* **2**, 891.

UNICEF and World Health Organization 1989: *Protecting, promoting and supporting breastfeeding; the special role of maternity services*. Geneva: World Health Organization.

United Kingdom Central Council for Nursing, Midwifery and Health Visiting 1992: *Code of professional conduct*. London: UKCC.

Walker, M. 1993: A fresh look at the risks of artificial infant feeding. *Journal of Human Lactation* **9**, 97–107.

Wallerstein, N. and Bernstein, E. 1988: Empowerment education: Freire's ideas adapted to health education. *Health Education Quarterly* **15**, 379–94.

White, A., Freeth, S. and O'Brien, M. 1992: *Infant Feeding 1990 Office of Population Censuses and Surveys*. London: HMSO.

Whitley, N. 1978: Preparation for breastfeeding: a one-year follow-up of 34 nursing mothers. *Journal of Obstetric, Gynaecologic and Neonatal Nursing* **7**, 44–8.

World Health Organization 1987: *International code of marketing of breastmilk substitutes*. Geneva: World Health Organization.

World Health Organization 1990: *Data bank on prevalence and duration of breastfeeding*. Geneva: Nutrition Unit, World Health Organization.

9

Empowerment for health: the challenge

Keith Tones

Sir, we know the will is free, and there's an end on't!

(Dr Samuel Johnson, 1709–1784)

The chapters in this book have provided a multitude of perspectives on empowerment in a variety of situations. It is apparent, however, that there is no readily available and universally agreed definition of empowerment; it is equally apparent that despite some definitional uncertainties, there is virtual unanimity that empowerment is good for health !

As was indicated in Chapter 3, if programmes designed to empower are to be efficiently designed and their effectiveness is to be demonstrated, the concept of empowerment must be operationalized and its implications opened up to scrutiny. In this chapter, the relationship between self-empowerment and community empowerment will be explored, together with the nature of the interaction between individuals, their environment and the power structure in which they work and live. The de-powering effects of the 'medical model' will be considered, and it will be argued that community participation is not only ideologically but also practically a *sine qua non* of effective and 'healthy' programmes. It will also be argued that the synergistic relationship between health education and *'healthy public policy'* should provide a basis for analysing and organizing community-based health promotion strategies. Education for individual empowerment, critical consciousness-raising and advocacy for social and organizational change should be the driving force behind the promotion of people's health.

Empowering communities

As was noted in Chapter 3, health choices are determined by the reciprocal relationship between individuals and their environment. Whether or not an

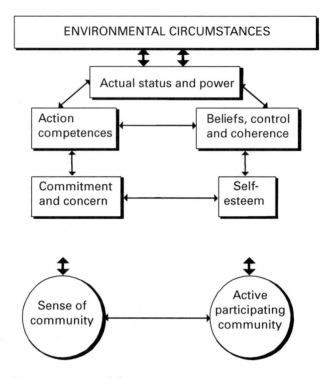

Figure 9.1 Empowerment and the environment

individual is free to choose depends substantially on whether the environment acts as a barrier to healthy choices. On the other hand, individuals may succeed in exerting an influence on their environments. The extent to which this is possible will, in turn, depend on the extent to which individuals are *self-empowered* and belong to *active participating communities.*

Figure 9.1 above represents this relationship between individual and community empowerment.

Reciprocal determinism: individual against environment?

The *reciprocal determinism* of environment and individual features prominently in Figure 9.1. The environment, of course, comprises a wide range of different circumstances. These may be physical, socio-economic and cultural. Roberts, in Chapter 6, clearly demonstrates the interaction of physical and socio-economic factors in the aetiology of accidents – poorer children are substantially more likely to be exposed to environmental hazards than their more fortunate middle-class counterparts. Again, the culture of poverty will limit capacity for healthy action and exacerbate the already existing negative effects of living in hazardous and generally squalid surroundings. (Empowered individuals will have a greater chance of changing their circumstances but those same circumstances will limit their opportunity for self-empowerment.)

Dynamics of self-empowerment

Reference was made in Chapter 3 to the potential contribution of self-empowerment to the making and sustaining of health actions. Some further brief observations on the dynamics of self-empowerment will be made here, in the context of the complex interrelationships between individuals, the communities in which they live and the all-embracing influence of environment. In short, self-empowerment involves the possession of a relatively high degree of control over one's life and circumstances, i.e. the possession of a relatively high degree of power and resources. (Self-empowerment is associated with certain beneficial psychological characteristics, prominent among which are beliefs about control and level of self-esteem) Beliefs about control are associated with self-esteem. Although self-esteem is substantially influenced by the way in which we are treated by other people – by, for example, whether we receive love and respect – it is also influenced by the amount of control we have or perceive that we have over our lives. Self-esteem is deemed to be intrinsically healthy (at least in western cultures) – e.g. as an important facet of mental health – and to contribute instrumentally to healthy choices. At the common-sense level, if we value ourselves we are more likely to respond to exhortations to look after ourselves!

As we shall see later, control is not a unitary concept and may vary in degree. Individuals may enjoy a high level of *internality* (i.e. they may believe that virtually whatever happens to them – good or bad – is due to their own initiative). *Externals*, on the other hand, tend to attribute such outcomes to the effects of outrageous fortune and/or to the influence of powerful others.

A more useful and practical notion deriving from Social Learning Theory (Bandura, 1982) is the concept of *self-efficacy*. Quite simply, if people do not believe they are capable of achieving a *specific* goal, they are unlikely to make the attempt, even though they might value the outcome. By contrast, the prognosis of a patient who has recently experienced heart surgery will be much better if he or she believes it is actually possible to adopt an accelerating programme of exercise without suffering a further heart attack or dropping dead from the effort. Arguably, the greater the number of specific, positive self-efficacy beliefs, the greater the perception of a relatively high degree of internal locus of control.

Salutogenesis and the sense of coherence

Antonovsky's theory of *salutogenesis* has a double relevance for health promotion. First, it emphasizes positive aspects of health and well-being and legitimizes a degree of deviation from a preventive medical model. Second, a key component of the theory – the *'sense of coherence'* – has particular relevance to the promotion of both mental and social health. The notion of coherence is compatible with the beliefs about control mentioned above, and indeed it adds an extra dimension. 'Salutogenesis' is, in Antonovsky's words, *'negentropic'*. In other words, coherence represents characteristics which help individuals to 'do battle with the entropic forces' which lead to chaos and meaninglessness (Antonovsky, 1984).

> The sense of coherence is '… a global orientation that expresses the extent to which one has a pervasive, enduring though dynamic feeling of confidence that one's internal and external environments are predictable and that there is a high probability that things will work out as well as can reasonably be expected.'
>
> (Antonovsky, 1984, p. 123)

The three main components of coherence are:

- *comprehensibility* – the world is 'ordered, consistent, structured and clear … and the future predictable' rather than 'noisy, chaotic, disordered, random, accidental and unpredictable';
- *manageability* – individuals believe that they have the kinds of resources at their disposal which will help them to manage their lives;
- *meaningfulness* – life makes sense emotionally; people are committed; they invest energy in worthwhile goals.

Clearly, the concept of manageability incorporates beliefs about control (e.g. internality or self-efficacy). Moreover, together with the idea of meaningfulness, it also includes those situations in which individuals are patently not in control, e.g. they may be terminally ill but they do not feel victimized because they believe that powerful others are *legitimately* in control, for example, 'friends, colleagues, God, history' (Antonovsky, 1984). This rather idiosyncratic interpretation of control is interestingly similar to Lewis' (1987) concept of *'existential control'*, which again refers to circumstances in which the individual does not exercise control but can impose meaning on his or her circumstances, and is thus relatively content.

While these latter notions may not be viewed as control in the normal sense of the word, they are highly significant in 'therapeutic' terms. Doubtless, the potential for conflict will not have escaped the reader! Consider those health promoters whose major goal is to generate indignation at social injustice and to empower individuals and communities so that they both believe they are capable of influencing their destiny and actively strive to do so. Imagine their dilemma when faced with individuals and communities who are not merely stoical in the face of ill health and adversity, but seem quite contented with their lot. In Panglossian terms, 'All is for the best in the best of all possible worlds!'

Returning to Figure 9.1 and the more orthodox conceptualization of control, one of the most important health promotion activities is to provide people with *'action competences'* or *'lifeskills'* (such as those provided by assertiveness training). The assumption, quite rightly, is that since nothing succeeds like success (in modifying beliefs about control and enhancing self-esteem) people should be provided with the skills that are needed to succeed.

Community empowerment

The meaning and dynamics of self-empowerment are reasonably clear. The notion of an empowered community is more contestable. For instance, is an empowered community merely the sum total of the empowered individuals who are members of that community? Certainly an empowered community will presumably be more likely to be mobilized in the pursuit of health and, generally, conform to the criteria of an *'active empowered community'* which received prominence in the Ottawa Charter. It will also contribute to individual empowerment both directly and indirectly via the processes of socialization.

On the other hand, there are those who argue that a *'sense of community'* is a central feature of a healthy, empowered community (Maton and Rappaport, 1984; Zimmerman, 1990). McMillan and Chavis (1986) have identified four main characteristics of a sense of community:

- *membership* – a feeling of belonging;
- *shared emotional connection* – 'the commitment and belief that members have shared and will share history, common places, time together, and similar experiences';
- *influence* – a sense of mattering;
- *integration and fulfilment of needs* – 'a feeling that members' needs will be met by the resources received through their membership in the group'.

The first three of the criteria bear an obvious similarity to the sense of coherence mentioned above. It seems highly likely that an individual who is a member of such a community might well be socialized into a degree of 'healthy' commitment and concern – provided, of course, that the community norms are consistent with such altruistic motives.

The fourth criterion also relates more directly to the empowerment dimension – provided that the community actually has genuine resources to offer, individuals might acquire the competences and confidence needed to tackle environmental constraints and generally to act in a proactive fashion. The extensive literature on social support provides additional justification for assertions about the benefits of a sense of community.

Although it is perhaps customary to think of a community as a geographically based group of lay people, all of the points discussed above have relevance for 'professional' communities such as hospitals. The significance of an empowering ethos in medical organizations has been discussed elsewhere in this book and needs no further comment here.

Power and its locus

It is certainly not original to point out that the issue of power and resources is central to the influence which environmental circumstances exert on individual choices (as shown in Figure 9.1). As we shall observe later, creating a sense of belonging and striving to energize and mobilize communities may well come to nothing if the issue of power is not fully addressed, since the distribution of power and wealth ultimately determines the possibilities of individual action. Indeed, a chapter in Ryan's (1976) classic text on victim-blaming is headed 'In Praise of Loot and Clout'. In it, Ryan quotes Fanny Brice, the vaudeville star, who reputedly said, 'I've been rich and I've been poor – and, believe me, rich is better!' Ryan's quite firm conviction about the social-structural roots of ill health and other social ills (rather than the individual and psychological) is revealed by the following vituperative quotation:

> Being poor is stressful. Being poor is worrisome; one is anxious about the next meal, the next dollar, the next day. Being poor is nerve-wracking, upsetting. When you're poor, its easy to despair and it's easy to lose your temper. And all of this is because you're poor. Not because your mother let you go around with your diapers full of a bowel movement until you were four, or shackled you to the potty chair before you could walk. Not because she broke your bottle on your first birthday or breast-fed you until you could cut your own steak. But because you don't have any *money*.
>
> (Ryan, 1976, p. 157)

However, we should not underestimate the power of cultural norms in either facilitating or impeding health choices. For instance, Gordon (Chapter 8) provides a nice description of an empowered breast-feeder ('a woman with a wild lot of confidence') – admittedly as viewed from the rather jaundiced eye of a disapproving partner! Clearly, while bottle-feeding was the 'norm', breastfeeding was not such a deviant activity that the breast-feeder would be completely ostracized (although she might have to carry out her somewhat deviant practices in private). Consider, however, the following description of the opposite scenario. Harfouche described the potential effect of socialization and normative pressure on women's feeding intentions in a particular Islamic culture:

> Lactation management and breastfeeding as an act and way of life are acquired in the home. The pattern has a familial transmission; girls usually identify with their mothers, and after marriage they try to comply with the wishes of their in-laws and husbands.
>
> (Harfouche, 1970)

Since breastfeeding was the norm, the social pressure on individual women to conform was clearly enormous. Breast milk was viewed as 'God's special gift to the infant. ... It is the best food and there is nothing like it.' As for the mother, 'Nursing is a duty; a mother who does not nurse denies her baby's right ... she is stingy, lazy, negligent, lacks affection like a stepmother. No lactation, no affection.'

While the situation described by Harfouche might be viewed by zealous paediatricians with considerable satisfaction, it is clearly fundamentally de-powering. Indeed, normative pressure has acted more efficiently than restrictive *healthy public policy* in making the healthy choice the only choice!

Reflections on medical dominance

In Chapter 3, the requirements for an empowering health-promoting encounter between health professional and client were identified. The approach in question is entirely consistent with Macleod Clark's (1993) notion of *'health nursing'* and Latter, in Chapter 1, provides a convincing demonstration of both success and failure in achieving the empowering interaction between nurse and patient. Interestingly, nurses on the 'de-powering' wards demonstrate similar 'top-down' behaviour as does the sample of health visitors interviewed by Kendall (1991). Latter provides convincing evidence that empowering encounters need empowered nurses, and notes the negative effects of the bureaucratized systems characteristic of hospitals – which, of course, have been used as classic exemplars of 'total institutions' (Taylor, 1979).

Despite stating the obvious, it is worth recalling that empowerment of both nurse and patient is problematical within the general context of medical hegemony. For this reason, the philosophy of health promotion incorporates both the importance of de-medicalizing health and de-mystifying medicine – and requires the reorientation of health services. The attack on medicine is not new. McKeown (1979), in his seminal critique of curative medicine, mischievously cites Nancy Mitford's comparison of medical practice in the time of Louis XIV with contemporary practice:

> In those days, terrifying in black robes and bonnets they bled the patient; now, terrifying in white robes and masks, they pump blood into him. The result is the same: the strong live; the weak, after much suffering and expense, both of spirit and money, die.
>
> (Mitford, 1969)

Kelleher *et al.* (1994) provide a more recent but similar thrust, noting that: 'the occupation of healing changed from being frequently seen as a rattlebag of quacks and rogues to a profession with considerable power, authority and status.'

While such challenges are doubtless gratifying and still have a degree of validity, it is more productive to consider some of the reasons for the existence of an imbalance of power between doctor and patient (and 'subordinate' professions allied to medicine) – other than those of sheer professional self-interest. A major reason for this differential in status and authority – with which many patients happily collude – is explicable by the classic formulation of the sick role (Parsons, 1951, 1979; Tones, 1998). This is sufficiently well known not to require reiteration here. However, let us recall that in return for legitimation of the sick role, patients have an obligation to seek medical help (for appropriate conditions) and to *comply with medical advice*. Compliance is quite clearly incompatible with autonomy, self-determination and empowerment. Moreover, and more specifically, the traditional doctor–patient relationship militates against the empathic and liberating techniques described in Chapter 3 and illustrated by Latter (see Chapter 1). Doctors (and therefore nurses) were expected to 'deny reciprocity' and to eschew this kind of relationship as DiMatteo and DiNicola (1982) observed: 'The disparity in power and control carves an emotional chasm between physician and patient – a chasm that is bridged only by the physician's altruism and orientation to serving people.'

Action for change: advocacy and healthy public policy

We turn now to a consideration of how health promotion might be expected to instigate change through empowerment. The first strategy reflects the first part of the 'formula' stating that health promotion involves healthy public policy multiplied by health education. As stated earlier, policy change might be achieved through lobbying and advocacy and/or through education. Policy initiatives operate at macro-, meso- and micro-levels: they involve, for example, legal measures at national or international level. Recent government proposals for banning all advertising and sponsorship of tobacco exemplifies a macro-level initiative of this kind. Organizational change operates at a meso-level. It might include a change in policy designed to meet the requirements of a *'health-promoting school'*. Policy levels do not act independently and, for instance, micro-level policy which provides training for ward nurses in active listening will be facilitated – or indeed may only be possible – within a *'health-promoting hospital'*.

Clearly those policies which address fundamental problems, such as poverty, will have a more substantial impact than micro-policies. For example, we quoted earlier Ryan's view that only radical social change could avoid accusations of victim-blaming. Galbraith (1992) also argues that the task facing countries such as North America and the UK is one of tackling the imbalance in power between the 'haves' and 'have-nots'. However, he emphasizes that national policy is necessary to tackle a *'culture of contentment'* in which an oppressed and de-powered underclass coexists with a majority of citizens who, in Macmillan's oft-quoted term, 'have never had it so good'.

> The present and devastated position of the . . . underclass has been identified as the most serious social problem of the time, as it is also the greatest threat to long-run peace and civility.

Life in the great cities in general could be improved, and only will be improved, by public action – by better schools with better paid teachers, by strong, well financed welfare services, by counseling on drug addiction, by employment training, by public investment in the housing that in no industrial country is provided for the poor by private enterprise, by adequately supported health care, recreational facilities, libraries and police. The question once again, much accommodating rhetoric to the contrary, is not what can be done but what will be paid.

(Galbraith, 1992)

While it is true that such dramatic and fundamental social policy change provides what is perhaps the ultimate solution to poor health and de-powerment, the magnitude of the task and the panic experienced by most governments at the financial costs involved render the prospect of action unlikely. It is important, therefore, to avoid the pessimistic view that *only* substantial policy change is worthy of action. Change can be achieved on a smaller scale, and Gordon (see Chapter 8) describes the implementation of a breastfeeding policy at organizational level which supports individual women's desire to follow their inclinations. Again at a more basic level, Kelleher *et al.* (1994) identified a number of diverse influences which have threatened the dominance of medicine. These include the challenge from an increasingly powerful management culture in the UK health service, the professionalization of professions allied to medicine – especially nursing, the increasing threat of litigation, the important influence of the feminist movement, the importance of some self-help groups and even the phenomenon of 'trial by television'.

Action for change: empowering communities

As has been noted previously, a central tenet of health promotion is the importance of community participation, not only because it is an integral part of the ethics of health promotion and health care but also because any kind of change is unlikely to occur or to be sustained unless people participate in the decision-making process. There are, of course, different degrees of participation, ranging from mere tokenism to autonomous decision-making, and Brager and Specht's (1973) spectrum of participation still offers one of the best typologies (see Figure 9.2).

Empowerment through community development

Community development (CD) is characterized by the seventh position in the typology in Figure 9.2. Its ethic and purpose are congruent with the radical imperative of those who argue that the first task of health promotion is to challenge *the culture of contentment* and to achieve a fairer balance of power and resources in society. An essential feature of CD is to generate

Degree of participation	Action	Nature of community involvement
LOW	None	I Community told nothing
	Receive information	II Organization makes plan and announces it. Community expected to comply
	Consulted	III Organization tries to promote plan and develop support in order to have it accepted
	Advises	IV Organization presents a plan and invites questions. Is prepared to modify plan only if absolutely necessary
	Plans jointly	V Organization presents a tentative plan subject to change and invites recommendations from those affected
	Has delegated authority	VI Organization identifies and presents a problem, defines the limits and asks the community to make a series of decisions to be embodied in a plan they will accept
	Has control	VII Organization asks the community to identify the problems and to make all the key decisions about ways and means. It is willing to help the community accomplish its own goals at each step, even to the extent of giving administrative control of the programme
HIGH		

Figure 9.2 A spectrum of participation

community participation, that is 'a process by which ordinary people can have some say in prioritising, planning, delivering and reviewing services' (UK Health For All Network, 1993).

Its approach is therefore fundamentally 'bottom-up'. Its purpose is to help a community to identify its 'felt needs' and then, through a process of empowerment, to provide support in order to help its members to satisfy the needs which they have identified. Their felt needs may, of course, not match the objectives established by health authorities – in fact it would be quite unusual if they were to do so. However, it is possible to adopt a quite radical empowering approach which maximizes participation while addressing issues which are the concern of preventive medicine. Rosenthal (1983) listed the characteristics of these 'community health projects' as follows:

- they are firmly based outside the health professions;
- they are concerned with addressing inequalities in health and health care provision;
- they are concerned to promote collective awareness of social causes of ill health;
- they assert that the monopoly of the information about health and ill health by professionals must be challenged both individually and collectively;
- activities centre on work with small groups of local people;
- projects have a catalyst function in stimulating local health, social and education services.

Roberts in Chapter 6 provides examples of such projects in the field of accident prevention.

Critical consciousness-raising and advocacy for action

As was observed in Chapter 3, health education has a dual function – empowering individual choices and raising consciousness about social and health issues so that, hopefully, healthy public policy may be implemented. The term 'critical consciousness-raising' (CCR) refers to the approach adopted by Freire (1972). This empowering process would ideally be applied to community development, and is summarized in Figure 9.3.

The consciousness-raising approach should not be limited to informal work in the community, and it is possible within the context of the health-promoting school to help young people to appraise critically social circumstances which militate against health. This could realistically involve, for example, a review of attempts by advertisers to manipulate food preferences, or close scrutiny of the statistics on inequalities in the distribution of health and illness – preferably with the full co-operation of mathematics teachers. We should perhaps not view these radical initiatives in the classroom as extraordinary – at least at a philosophical level. It could be argued that a radical and critically questioning approach to society is the central purpose of education. Indeed, Scambler and Scambler, in Chapter 5, have drawn our attention to the importance to 'Civil Society' of 'an open and egalitarian consideration of contemporary issues'. The specific 'matter for public deliberation' was, in that case, the empowerment of women sex workers.

The Scamblers' chapter also cautions us against making premature judgements in their challenge to the common-sense notion that sex workers

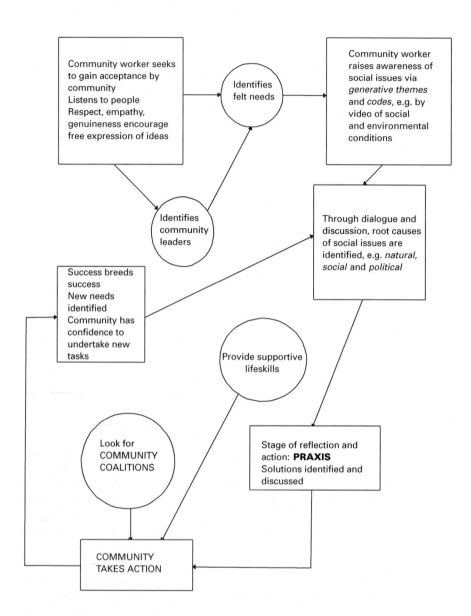

Figure 9.3 Critical consciousness-raising and community action. Actions in circles are additions to the Freirean approach

are necessarily de-powered. They demonstrated quite convincingly that at least some workers are in control of their lives and appear to have made a conscious decision to adopt their chosen career. That chapter also exemplifies the advocacy function in its comments on the contribution of the English Collective of Prostitutes. None the less, Scambler and Scambler also point out the need to reorient health services in order to provide the necessary support, and they emphasized the fact that the recruitment of many workers was essentially non-voluntary.

Problems for community development

Despite its apparent position on the moral high ground, community development is open to criticism. For example, Constantino-David (1982), among other criticisms, cautioned against the community becoming dependent on community workers. She warned against creating a new elite from community aides or indigenous workers, and she commented on the frustration of change agents who wished to address the fundamental problems of inequalities but had first to work through the community's felt needs which, although they might fire people's imagination, might be insignificant in the longer term. She also identified a kind of pseudo-empowerment resulting from a process she termed *'facipulation'*, whereby the change agent appeared to facilitate the achievement of community goals, but in reality manipulated the agenda and steered people towards issues which the change agent considered to be important.

A particular problem derives from the often inevitable tension between health service managers' concerns and perspectives, and the concerns and perspectives of the community and the community workers. Even if the managers understand and acknowledge the importance of horizontal programmes (see Chapter 3), the political imperative and government epidemiologically based targets may preclude any official engagement in CD or the provision of financial support. Accordingly, community health projects have to survive on short-term funding, and many a project collapses when the money runs out – presumably leaving the community more disillusioned than it was at the beginning of the programme. A related and more powerful argument against CD derives from the conviction that there is a limit to the extent to which disadvantaged communities can empower themselves in the context of an oppressive regime. CD projects can thus be neatly integrated within a dominant, top-down ideology, since there is little genuine threat to the system.

The process of critical consciousness-raising itself may not only be ineffective but even hazardous – as many disenfranchized peasants and health service 'whistleblowers' have learned to their cost! Accordingly, two principles must guide those who engage in consciousness-raising.

- Never raise consciousness without providing supportive lifeskills which help people to achieve true praxis by translating indignation into effective practice.
- Give careful thought to the aftermath and adopt the 'ostrich position' – don't bury your head in the sand, but take care before you stick it over the parapet!

The case for coalitions

Because of the limitations inherent in CD, two major kinds of alternative to creating community change have been proposed. The first of these consists of more direct and radical *social action* involving confrontation and protest – and stopping just short of revolution. It is archetypically associated with Saul Alinksy (Alinsky, 1946). The second and much more respectable strategy involves the development of *community coalitions*. It is argued that change is more likely to happen if coalitions of those having status, resources and power are formed to combat the substantial influence of government, commercial and other vested interests (Goodman *et al.*, 1993). Community participation is considered to be an essential feature of successful coalitions, often in the form of *citizen boards*. Unfortunately, the probability of the kinds of tokenism outlined in Brager and Specht's continuum must be relatively high.

Media advocacy

It is probably unusual to introduce the mass media into a discussion about empowerment for health since, traditionally, the function of mass media has been to persuade, cajole and manipulate in an attempt to market health, often in a blatant top-down fashion. Although further discussion is beyond the scope of this chapter, it is important to signal the potentially powerful strategy of *media advocacy* (for further discussion, see Chapman and Lupton, 1994; Tones, 1996). In short, media advocacy utilizes what is potentially the most powerful function of mass media – to raise awareness. This agenda-setting function is often enhanced by the use of *'creative epidemiology'*, namely the presentation of health data in a dramatic and shocking form. The purpose is to create healthy public policy. As with community coalitions, programmes are typically vertical (e.g. smoking or the prevention of heart disease) rather than horizontal (e.g. seeking to generate public outrage at the increasing gap in health between the rich and the poor).

Thoughts on empowering the elderly

It is commonplace in preventive medicine and health promotion to identify at-risk groups. It is equally sensible to identify those groups of individuals who are de-powered and therefore merit particular consideration. We have already commented on the needs of the 'underclass', and communities experiencing multiple disadvantage and other deprived groups have been readily identified. These latter groups include various ethnic minorities and, globally, women in general. Before concluding the chapter, a few comments will be made about the needs of older people.

In many cultures and societies, the elderly are likely to be one of the least empowered categories of citizens – partly due to relative poverty and partly due to cultural expectations and stereotyping.

Healthy communication with the elderly

Three kinds of health action will be mentioned here, and the first of these derives from Le May's observations about the importance of empowering older people through communication (see Chapter 4). We merely need to reiterate earlier assertions that the first important contribution to empowering individuals involves active listening and the kind of interpersonal encounter discussed in Chapter 3.

Creating a positive image of ageing

A second approach seeks to provide a community-wide approach to *'building a positive image of ageing'*, which involves the kind of coalition-building that was discussed earlier in this chapter. Kemper and Mettler (1990) describe a programme in Boise, Idaho – a city with a population of 102,000 people. A non-profit-making health promotion organization (*'Healthwise'*) acted as a lead agency with the local Council on Aging and built a coalition which included local workplaces, schools, the YMCA and YWCA, two hospitals, the University and the District Health Department. A high level of participation by older people themselves was achieved and committees were formed from local senior citizens' groups. A *'Growing Younger'* workshop programme was initiated, which focused on:

- improving flexibility, strength and endurance;
- improving diet;
- relieving stress and muscle tension;
- improving the quality of care received at home and from the participants' doctors.

We should note that although the workshop topics seem to be mainly concerned with an individual preventive medical model, the discovery that it was possible to achieve change clearly influenced a number of self-efficacy beliefs and generated greater self-confidence.

The programme apparently expanded considerably and *'Growing Younger'* subsequently developed a *'Growing Wiser'* mental health programme.

During the first 30 months, 1658 older adults (12 per cent of the over-60s population) participated in the programme. During an 18-month evaluation period, some 578 senior citizens participated in the *'Growing Wiser'* campaign, with an average age of 71 years. Apart from demonstrable changes in physical and mental health status at the individual level (e.g. a 24 per cent improvement in the risk of geriatric depression), the Boise experience had a quite dramatic effect on building healthy public policy. At a local level, changes were made in the organization of senior citizen centres, and older people lobbied the Area Agency on Aging and achieved a change in the provision of meals services. The regional medical centre expanded its services for the elderly and created a new Senior Life Center to meet their needs.

The success of the project generated widespread interest and resulted in substantial additional state funding. Moreover, the state adopted the approach and principles of the Boise project and, according to the authors, similar programmes were established in over 100 communities in 30 states nationwide.

A supportive environment in a nursing home

The high level of citizen involvement in the Boise Project reminds us of the potentially substantially *real power* exercised by the elderly. Although militant wings of older people – such as the *Grey Panthers* – have adopted a radical campaigning approach for old people's rights, it is important to recall that elderly people are not a minority group. Indeed their numbers increase yearly, much to the consternation of governments which are horrified at the prospect of the pensions bill! If in fact a new image of ageing can be created and older people can be more empowered, they might have a substantial effect merely through using the ballot box.

It is, of course, now recognized that such a large group of citizens cannot merely be classified as old. At the very least we should identify two categories – the 'young old', many of whom will have occupational pensions and be financially secure, and the 'frail elderly'. While campaigning might well be appropriate for the younger group, the frail elderly cannot be neglected. The third example of empowerment therefore refers to such a group, and illustrates the combined effects of healthy public policy in providing a supportive environment as a background to providing care and communication.

Langer and Rodin (1976) deliberately set out to enhance the independence and personal control of a group of elderly people in a nursing home. Within the nursing home, residents were randomly assigned to an experimental condition and a control condition. The home was described by the researchers as 'modern' and of high quality. There were already a number of opportunities to influence the ways in which the home was run, e.g. by influencing the menus. However, the experimental group was counselled about these various opportunities and encouraged to use them. More importantly, they were invited to decide how the furniture in their rooms should be arranged, and were given potted plants *to look after*. The control group, which occupied a different but similar floor in the home, was merely given the plants – which were cared for by the nursing staff. Measures of activity levels and general happiness were recorded, and there was a significant difference in the quality of life of the 'responsibility' group. They were more active, alert and contented than their counterparts. In Antonovsky's terms, they presumably had a greater sense of coherence. However, one of the most interesting features of this research was the apparent improvement in physical health of the 'empowered' elderly group compared to the controls, whose death rate over the following months was twice that of the frail elderly who had acquired some degree of control over their lives.

Participation and community change

Classic Communication of Innovations Theory identifies key influences on the likelihood of communities adopting innovations. These include people's perceptions of the characteristic of the innovation in question. For instance, if they consider that breastfeeding involves a good deal of aggravation while apparently conveying few benefits, its adoption will at worst never happen, and at best take a long time.

There is, however, a general precept about the likelihood of change, and this centres on that central concept which has been emphasized in this and other chapters in the book – namely participation. Figure 9.4 shows how the chances of adopting any new ideas or practices will depend on two variables: (i) who determines the need and (ii) who provides the solution to the problem associated with the needs assessment exercise.

Briefly, when the community itself recognizes that it has a problem and identifies its own need – and creates its own solution to that problem, change will be rapid. Indeed, no intervention will be necessary from outside organizations, health services or individual health personnel: change will just happen.

On the other hand, when professionals identify the need or problem and decide to intervene and then impose the solution on a bemused community, change will occur very slowly or else not at all.

However, if a 'change agent' such as a health worker works gently and empathetically with the community, making every encounter an empowering one, the community itself may come to identify its needs. If the change agent then uses the same techniques to help the community to discover ways of meeting those needs, change may very well happen. It may not happen very quickly, but the change is likely to be enduring, as it has passed into community ownership.

The situation is nicely described by a frequently quoted poem – reputedly of Chinese origin:

Extent of community involvement	Anticipated rate of adoption of innovation
Community spontaneously recognizes it has a problem Community identifies solution to problem	RAPID ADOPTION
External agency considers that community has a problem Prescribes solution	VERY SLOW – OR NEVER!

Figure 9.4 Extent of community participation and the likelihood of action

Go to the people
Love them
Start with what they know
Build on what they have
But of the best leaders
When their task is accomplished
Their work is done
The people all remark
We have done it ourselves.

(Chabot, 1976)

References

Alinsky, S.D. 1946: *Reveille for Radicals*. New York: Vintage Books.
Antonovsky, A. 1984: The sense of coherence as a determinant of health. In Matarazzo, J.D., Weiss, S.M., Herd, J.A. *et al.* (eds), *Behavioral health*. New York: John Wiley, 114–29.

Bandura, A. 1982: Self-efficacy mechanism in human agency. *American Psychologist* **37**, 122–47.

Brager, C. and Specht, H. 1973: *Community organising*. Columbia, NY: Columbia University Press.

Chabot, J.H.T. 1976: The Chinese system of health care. *Tropical Geographical Medicine* **28**, 87–134.

Chapman, S. and Lupton, D. 1994: *The fight for public health: principles and practice of media advocacy*. London: BMJ Publications.

Constantino-David, K. 1982: Issues in community organization. *Community Development Journal* **17**, 190–201.

DiMatteo, M.R. and DiNicola D.D. 1982: *Achieving patient compliance: the psychology of the medical practitioner's role*. New York: Pergamon.

Freire, P. 1972: *Pedagogy of the oppressed*. London: Sheed and Ward.

Galbraith, J.K. 1992: *The culture of contentment*. Harmondsworth: Penguin.

Goodman, R.M., Burdine, J.N., Meehan, E. and McLeroy, K.R. 1993: Special issue on community coalitions. *Health Education Research: Theory and Practice* **8**, 122–31.

Harfouche, J.K. 1970: The importance of breast feeding. *Journal of Tropical Paediatrics* **16** (Monograph 10), 133–75.

Kelleher, D. Gabe, J. and Williams, G. 1994: Understanding medical dominance in the modern world. In Gabe, J., Kelleher, D. and Williams, G. (eds), *Challenging medicine*. London: Routledge. xi–xxix.

Kemper, D.W. and Mettler, M. 1990: Building a positive image of ageing: the experience of a small American city. In Bracht N. (ed.), *Health promotion at the community level*. Sage: Newbury Park.

Kendall, S. 1991: *An analysis of the health visitor–client interaction: the influence of the health visiting process on client participation*. Unpublished PhD Thesis, King's College, University of London, London.

Langer, E.J. and Rodin, J. 1976: The effects of enhanced personal responsibility for the aged. *Journal of Personality and Social Psychology*, **34**, 191–8.

Lewis, F.M. 1987: The concept of control: a typology and health related variables. *Advances in Health Education and Promotion* **2**, 277–309.

McKeown, T. 1979: *The role of medicine: dream, mirage or nemesis?* Oxford: Basil Blackwell.

Macleod Clark, J. 1993: From sick nursing to health nursing: evolution or revolution? In Wilson-Barnett, J. and Macleod Clark, J. (eds), *Research in health promotion and nursing*. Basingstoke: Macmillan Press, 256–70.

McMillan, D.W. and Chavis, D.M. 1986: Sense of community: a definition and theory. *Journal of Community Psychology* **14**, 6–23.

Maton, K.I. and Rappaport, J. 1984: Empowerment in a religious setting: a multivariate investigation. In Rappaport, J., Swift, C. and Hess, R. (eds), *Studies in empowerment: steps toward understanding and action*. New York: Haworth Press.

Mitford, N. 1969: *The sun king*. London: Sphere Books.

Parsons, T. 1951: *The social system*. New York: Free Press.

Parsons, T. 1979: Definitions of health and illness in the light of American values and social structure. In Jaco, E.G. (ed.), *Patients, physicians and illness*, 3rd edn. New York: Free Press, 120–44.

Rosenthal, H. 1983: Neighbourhood health projects: some new approaches to health and community work in parts of the United Kingdom. *Community Development Journal* **13**, 122–31.

Ryan, W. 1976: *Blaming the victim*. New York: Vintage Books.

Taylor, S.E. 1979: Hospital patient behavior: reactance, helplessness, or control? *Journal of Social Issues* **35**, 156–84.

Tones, B.K. 1996: Models of mass media: hypodermic, aerosol or agent provocateur? *Drugs: Education, Prevention and Policy* **3**, 29–37.

Tones, B.K. 1998: Health promotion: empowering choice. In Myers, L.B. and Midence, K. (eds), *Adherence to treatment in medical conditions*. Amsterdam: Harwood Academic, 133–60.

UK Health for All Network 1993: *Health for All resource pack*. Sheffield: District Health Authority.

Zimmerman, M.A. 1990: Toward a theory of learned hopefulness: a structural model analysis of participation and empowerment. *Journal of Research in Personality* **24**, 71–86.

Index